The

1   **The Current Position**

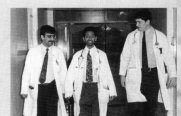

2   **Skill Mix and Deployment**

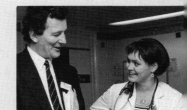

3   **The Contribution of Consultants**

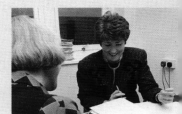

4   **The Organisation and Management of Training**

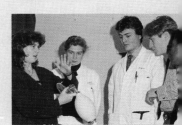

5   **A Framework for Change**

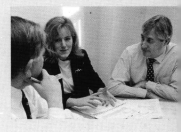

Contents

Preface 3

Introduction 4

1   **The Current Position** 7

Changing demand for health care and medical inputs 11

Changing supply of doctors 12

The local structure of medical staffing in the 1990s 14

2   **Skill Mix and Deployment** 16

The problems 17

Lack of clarity of what doctors should do 17

Insufficient supervision of junior doctors 20

Demand is seldom allocated or managed 23

Workload and staff availability are poorly matched 23

Many doctors feel unsupported in their work 24

Overcoming the problems 26

Define doctors' roles in relation to other professions 26

Clarify the allocation of tasks and supervision 28

Manage demand 28

Deploy doctors according to the demand 30

Provide better employment opportunities and support 32

Conclusion 33

Recommendations on skill mix and deployment 35

3   **The Contribution of Consultants** 37

The problems 38

Inadequate use of job plans 38

Variation in consultants' workloads 40

Overcoming the problems 45

Better use of job plans 45

More even distribution of the work 47

Recommendations for NHS trusts on the contribution of consultants 48

4   **The Organisation and Management of Training** 49

The problems 51

Inadequate management of postgraduate training 51

Inflexible training structures 54

Lack of professional development for career grade staff 55

Overcoming the problems 56

Improving the management of post graduate training 56

Providing more flexible training 58

Continuing professional development 59

Recommendations on the organisation and management of training 60

5   **A Framework for Change** 61

Appropriate national controls on medical staffing 62

Incentives for doctors at all levels 62

Clearer and more positive relationships between doctors and managers 64

Action checklist 66

Appendix 1 – Acknowledgements 68

The study sites 68

The advisory group 68

Appendix 2 – The Study Sites 70

Appendix 3 – Questionnaires Sent to Doctors at the Study Sites 71

Appendix 4 – NHS Operating Theatre Work 73

The sample 73

Data analysis 73

Results 74

Appendix 5 – Comparison of NHS and Private Operating Theatre Work 82

Appendix 6 – Consultants' NHS Outpatient Work 84

References 88

Index 91

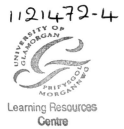
© Crown Copyright 1995
Application for reproduction should be made to HMSO

Printed in the UK for the Audit Commission at Stephens & George, Wales
ISBN 011 886 149 2
London: HMSO

Photographs by Hilary Shedel and with thanks to the staff of Kingston Hospital NHS Trust

Preface

The Audit Commission oversees the external audit of local authorities and agencies within the National Health Service (NHS) in England and Wales. As part of its function the Commission is charged with reviewing the economy, efficiency and effectiveness of services provided by those bodies. To this end, studies and audits of selected topics are undertaken each year.

This study of hospital medical staffing is concerned with the organisation and working practices of doctors in acute hospitals. It was carried out at various study sites across the country. A list of sites and details of the study methodology are given in the appendices. Local audits are now underway and will be carried out in all acute hospitals in England and Wales during the next year or so. The Audit Commission will be collecting more information from these audits along the lines of that set out in this report and aims to publish it as soon as possible.

The study was carried out by John Bailey, David Bawden, Dr Paul Baker and Paul Smith under the general direction of Dr Jonathan Boyce and Dr Jocelyn Cornwell. Kirti Patel and Dr James Gray assisted with data collection and analysis. Dr Robin Dowie (health services researcher) and David Ralphs (consultant surgeon) provided additional advice. The study was also supported by an advisory group (Appendix 1). The Audit Commission is grateful to all the individuals and organisations who assisted with this study. Responsibility for the contents and conclusions rests solely with the Audit Commission.

Introduction

'Many working practices derive from before the formation of the NHS and are now being rendered inappropriate by the changing environment'

1. Hospital doctors are central to the delivery of high quality patient care. They are the most important determinant of what a hospital does and consequently its use of resources. Doctors are also a significant resource in their own right. They deliver a substantial part of services, represent a major investment in training and skills and account directly for £2,000m of NHS expenditure – typically 14 per cent of an acute hospital budget. For all these reasons it is essential that doctors are properly supported in their work, and that they behave as committed and integral players in NHS trusts.

2. These reasons alone would be sufficient to justify a study of hospital medical staffing, but there are more. All hospital staff, and especially doctors, are currently being affected worldwide by major changes in health care. New technology has increased the scope of effective interventions to the point where more is on offer than we can conceivably afford. Whatever the health care system, those who hold the purse strings are increasingly having to determine their priorities and seek greater influence over the delivery of health care.

3. Doctors in the UK are facing even more changes, including:

◆ increasingly autonomous hospital management (trusts now hold contracts with their consultants and can vary terms and conditions of new posts);

◆ a more structured approach to medical training with a reduction in the time it takes to train as a specialist;

◆ strands of government policy that aim to:
a) increase the share of patient care provided by fully trained specialists;
b) reduce the long hours worked by many junior doctors.

4. These changes are a major challenge to hospitals and their doctors. Their main responsibility is to continue to provide the current high standard of patient care. Trusts must ensure that they provide sufficient doctors with appropriate skills when and where necessary. And because the NHS is a monopoly employer, it has a second clear responsibility to provide high quality training in its trusts. In fact, the training of young doctors can be improved considerably, and there is an urgent need to make training equally available to those who wish to train while working part-time. Structured and systematic continuing education for those who are fully trained is now accepted as necessary and desirable and must be properly provided by trusts.

5. If these responsibilities are to be discharged successfully, change will be necessary at a variety of levels, including the working practices of doctors and other professionals. Many working practices derive from before the formation of the NHS and are now being rendered inappropriate by the changing environment. Some doctors are already examining the details of the way they work, asking themselves where they ought to change and developing workable solutions. Doctors need to lead and shape the inevitable change in health care, rather than just reacting to it (Ref. 1).

6. Doctors will do this more easily and to best effect when they and managers work together on a common agenda. The traditional view of service issues as the province of managers, with patient care and medical training as the province of doctors is no longer tenable. Managers must take a share of the responsibility for patient care and medical training, at least by seeing that clinical professionals are well supported. Doctors for their part need to take more responsibility for the service as whole, their use of resources and the organisation and management of their own day-to-day work.

7. The agenda for change in the way doctors work, train and interact with the rest of the hospital is huge. Many aspects of it are extremely complex and sensitive. Yet if the problems can be tackled constructively, there are great benefits to be had. Not only can patient care be improved, but doctors should be able to do their jobs better and with greater satisfaction. This report aims to help identify and illuminate both the problems that have to be faced and wherever possible to suggest solutions. It contains a number of examples of good practice where positive action has already been taken to improve care processes and training. Equally, as the reader will see, it contains evidence of outmoded practices that must now change as a matter of urgency. The report is written primarily for clinical directors and consultants who are the main agents of change, but it is also aimed at senior trust managers, junior doctors and members of trust boards who also have important roles to play. Some of the recommendations are addressed to the Government and the medical royal colleges and their faculties.

8. The remainder of the report is structured as follows:

Chapter 1 sets out some current facts about medical staffing in England and Wales and the national context in which trusts must now work.

Chapter 2 looks at the deployment of doctors in relation to the demand and recommends better matching of the two in conjunction with greater clarity of doctors' roles and tasks.

Chapter 3 deals with consultants' contributions to the work of the hospital and argues that workloads should be more evenly distributed between them.

Chapter 4 looks at the local organisation of medical training and recommends a much more structured approach at all levels from the trust board to individual doctors.

Finally, **Chapter 5** looks at the main obstacles likely to impede change on these fronts and foresees changes in the national controls on medical staffing and the management structure and process in which doctors work.

9. This report has not covered all aspects of medical staffing. Some were impossible to research within the timescale of the study because of the paucity of good information. These include selection of doctors (e.g. statutory appointment committees for consultants) and disciplinary procedures. These issues will need to be examined in due course, and the Audit Commission will do so when time and resources allow. Other suggestions for work on medical staffing would, in the meantime, be welcomed.

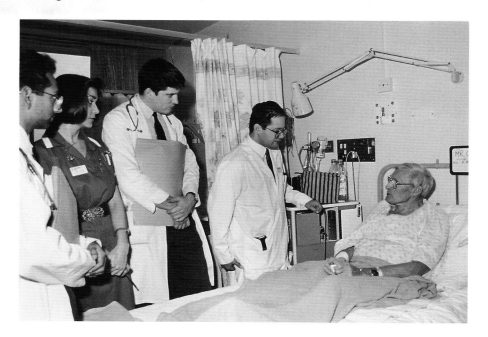

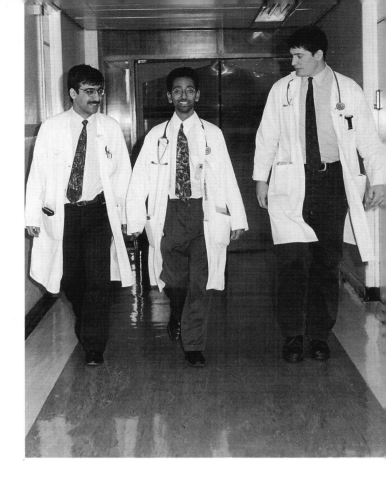

Demand for health care has been growing and so has the demand for doctors. Their work has become more intense and more specialised. The supply of doctors to the NHS has been dominated by several government initiatives aimed at increasing both the number of doctors and the share of work done by fully trained staff. Despite these pressures, doctors' working practices have stayed much the same and are now inappropriate for the context in which they work.

1 The Current Position

10. There are currently about 55,000 doctors working in hospitals in England and Wales. A district general hospital (DGH) typically has 170 doctors consisting of 70 consultants, 90 in the training grades (senior registrar, registrar, senior house officer and house officer, all undertaking postgraduate training) and ten in non-consultant career grades (associate specialist and staff grade). In addition, it may employ hospital practitioners and clinical assistants – who usually work primarily as GPs – for a small number of sessions per week, particularly in obstetrics, anaesthetics and accident and emergency (A & E). Hospital doctors in training grades are usually described as junior doctors, although they may have been qualified for as many as 15 years.

11. The hospital career ladder is long (Exhibit 1). At senior house officer level and below, hospitals provide general professional training for doctors who intend to become GPs or move into public health and other non-hospital grades as well as for those intending to pursue a hospital specialty. About 42 per cent of doctors remain in hospital medicine (mostly as consultants) and a third become GPs. The percentage becoming GPs is increasing as the number of posts in 'other NHS medicine' (mainly in community health) declines. Very few leave medicine altogether (Exhibit 2).

Exhibit 1
The hospital career ladder

The hospital career ladder is long.

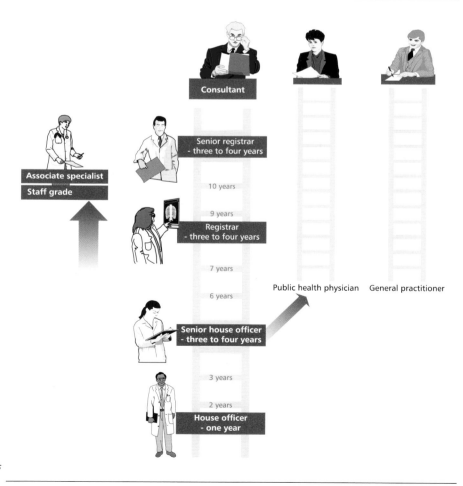

Source: Audit Commission (data on number of years in training grades from Ref. 2).

Exhibit 2
Posts achieved by doctors in 1986 who qualified from British medical schools in 1966

About 42 per cent of doctors remain in hospital medicine and a third become GPs.

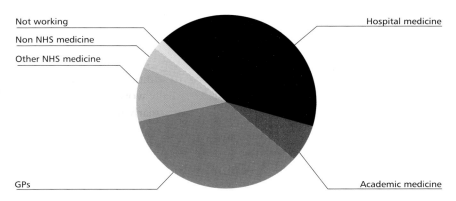

Source: Ref. 2.

12. Most hospital doctors work in the general medical and general surgical specialty groupings and in obstetrics and gynaecology, anaesthetics and paediatrics[1]. The general medical specialty grouping includes cardiology and nephrology, for example, as well as general medicine (Exhibit 3, overleaf). Similarly, the general surgical grouping includes orthopaedics and otolaryngology, for example, as well as general surgery.

13. The specialties differ in:

◆ the **ratio of trainees to consultants.** It varies from 1:1 in anaesthetics to 2.5:1 in obstetrics and gynaecology (Exhibit 4, overleaf).

◆ the **extent of emergency work**. In general medicine, general surgery, obstetrics and gynaecology, paediatrics and anaesthetics there is a high proportion of emergency work. In contrast, specialties such as otolaryngology or dermatology have a much lower emergency workload.

14. In recent years major changes have been taking place in the demand for and supply of doctors. This chapter examines the changes and discusses their effects on the local organisation of medical staffing.

[1]
Much of the detailed work in this report relates only to general medicine, general surgery, otolaryngology, trauma and orthopaedics, urology, anaesthetics and obstetrics and gynaecology, which alone account for 48 per cent of the hospital medical workforce. Doctors working in accident and emergency, radiology and pathology have been or are currently being included in other Audit Commission studies.

Exhibit 3
The distribution of hospital doctors by specialty in England and Wales, September 1993

Almost half of hospital doctors work in the general medical and general surgical specialty groupings.

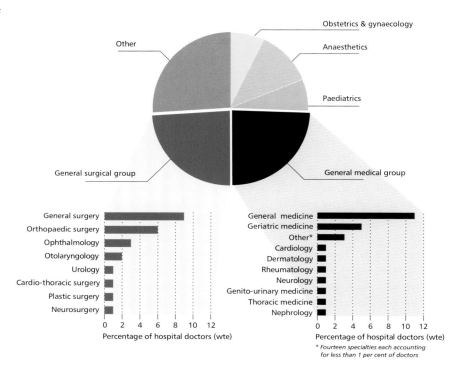

Note: The number of doctors is measured in whole-time equivalents (wtes). Hospital practitioners and clinical assistants are excluded.

Source: Department of Health Medical Manpower Statistics.

Exhibit 4
The ratio of trainees to consultants in the large specialties in England and Wales, September 1993

The ratio of trainees to consultants varies from 1:1 (anaesthetics) to 2.5:1 (obstetrics and gynaecology).

Note: Excludes house officers who work only in a few specialties and are not fully registered doctors.

Source: Department of Health Medical Manpower Statistics.

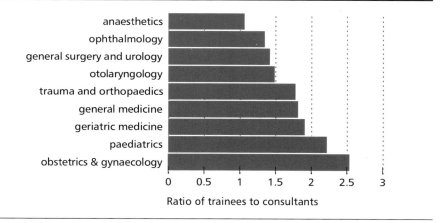

Changing demand for health care and medical inputs

15. The demand for health care has been growing steadily at least since the NHS was established in 1948. The number of inpatients, for example, has grown at about 2.3 per cent per year (1948-1992). More recently there has been a dramatic growth in day-case activity (an average of nine per cent per year in the past ten years and nearly twice this in 1992/93 to 1993/94). Day cases now account for a third of all surgical admissions to hospital.

16. A large part of the increase in demand is due to changes in the population and patterns of disease:

♦ The elderly population is growing. In particular, the number of people aged over 75 years has grown at two per cent per year since 1961, compared to 0.3 per cent per year for the population as a whole over the same period. Elderly people have consistently greater demand for health care than their younger counterparts.

♦ Diseases such as cancer and ischaemic heart disease are age related and so have become more common. Other diseases are relatively new (e.g. AIDS), are increasing in true incidence (e.g. malignant melanoma) or are on the wane (e.g. pneumonia).

17. In the past 20 years these demands have been met to some extent by an increase in the number of doctors (3.1 per cent per year). Indeed, the number of patients per doctor has fallen in the main specialties. However, as a measure of doctors' productivity this is too simplistic:

♦ Advances in medical technology and changes in disease management have indicated the scope and complexity of medical intervention. This is evidenced by growing specialisation in the medical workforce. In 1858 (the year the General Medical Council (GMC) was formed) there were three types of doctor: physicians, surgeons and apothecaries – the antecedents of GPs. Today the Department of Health collects medical workforce data on 55 specialties. Most of the growth in the number of acute specialties has taken place within the last 40 years (Exhibit 5).

♦ Patients now spend much less time in hospital. The average length of stay has fallen by 3.7 per cent per year since 1951, although they now often require more input from doctors, rather than less.

Exhibit 5
The growth in the number of acute specialties recognised by the Department of Health

The number of separate specialties has increased rapidly over recent years.

Note: Excludes pathology, radiology and psychiatric specialties.

Source: Ref. 3 (1859 and 1905); Department of Health Annual Reports and Health Statistics publications (1949 onwards).

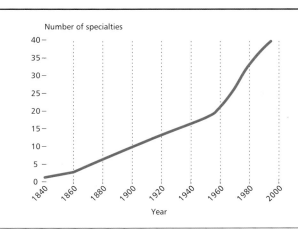

◆ Doctors' availability for patient care has diminished because they are increasingly expected to become involved in a variety of new activities such as clinical audit, negotiating with purchasers, developing new services and management.

Changing supply of doctors

18. The increase in demand and the necessary growth in the number of doctors have put stresses on the structure, conditions and training of the medical workforce. The supply of doctors has been dominated by several government initiatives on medical staffing and associated standards and rules in relation to training which involve several bodies including the GMC, universities and royal colleges.

19. Since 1987 the overall aim of national medical staffing policy has been:

'...to continue to improve the quality of patient services by increasing the level of service provided by fully trained doctors and by improving the standards of medical education and training' (Ref. 4).

There are three main government initiatives:

◆ *Achieving a Balance* in the grade structure of hospital doctors;

◆ the *New Deal* for junior doctors;

◆ the *Calman Report* on training.

'Achieving a Balance'

20. The main objective of *Achieving a Balance* (which was published in 1987) is to increase the number of career grade doctors relative to the number in training in order to improve the career prospects of those in training while still providing adequate support staff for consultants (Ref. 5). Doctors take, on average, 12 years after qualification from university to obtain a consultant post (Exhibit 1, page 8). *Achieving a Balance* aims to reduce this and to provide a smoother transition from training to career grades by:

◆ increasing the number of consultant posts;

◆ restricting the number of training posts; and

◆ introducing a new staff grade career post for doctors who do not wish or are unable to progress to the consultant grade.

21. *Achieving a Balance* projected an increase in the share of consultants in the medical workforce from 38 per cent in 1987 to 42 per cent in 1993 and a corresponding reduction in the share of the training grades. In practice, the planned growth of two per cent per year in the number of consultants has been achieved, but the share of consultants has remained almost constant and the share of training grades has gone down only slightly (Exhibit 6). Consultant posts tend to create more clinical work. Unless this growth in clinical work is controlled or consultants are prepared to take on all aspects of this work, including that traditionally carried out by juniors, there is a pressure to increase the number of junior posts at the same time, and the net effect naturally is that the ratio of trainees to consultants does not change.

Exhibit 6
Projected and actual changes in the grade structure of hospital doctors in England and Wales, 1987-1993

The share of consultants has remained almost constant and that of training grades has fallen only slightly.

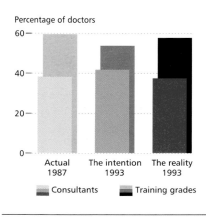

Percentage of doctors

Source: Ref. 5 and Department of Health Medical Manpower Statistics.

The 'New Deal'

22. The primary objective of the *New Deal* (which was published in 1991) is to reduce the long hours worked by many junior doctors (Ref. 6). It:

- sets firm limits on contracted hours (72 per week or less in most hospital posts) and working hours (56 per week) to be achieved in all hospitals;
- calls for a further increase in the number of consultant posts;
- encourages new ways of organising junior doctors' work such as shifts, partial shifts and cross-cover between specialties; and,
- seeks to improve facilities – such as residential accommodation and catering services – for junior doctors.

23. Its main achievements so far have been a reduction of 19 per cent in average contracted hours (including on-call duties) and of nine per cent in average working hours over the same period (Exhibit 7). Without more fundamental changes in the way doctors work and medical training is managed, trusts are likely to find it much more difficult to meet the more stringent requirements on hours which came into being in January 1995. The *New Deal* will force trusts to consider many of the issues raised in this report and the forthcoming local audits should assist them in doing so.

The Calman report

24. *Hospital Doctors: Training for the Future* the Calman report (published in 1993, Ref. 9) aims to bring the UK into line with other European Union (EU) countries in the definition of 'specialist' by reducing the length of doctors' postgraduate training. It seeks to:

- reduce the minimum length of postgraduate specialist training to seven years;
- introduce more explicit training curricula and a new Certificate of Completion of Specialist Training (CCST) to make it clear when training is complete; and
- merge the registrar and senior registrar grades to smooth the passage between the two grades.

It is too soon to judge the effects of the report, but there is little doubt that medical training is on the verge of a major change in direction, driven largely by the royal colleges. The proposals of more structured training and explicit

Exhibit 7
Recent changes in junior doctors' hours of work

Hours of contracted work have fallen, but the fall in hours actually worked has been less.

Average number of hours per week:	1987/88	1993	% change
contracted (including on-call hours)	90	73	-19
worked (including call-out hours)	58	53	-9

Source: Ref. 7 (1987/88), Ref. 8 (1993).

statements of a doctor's progress are revolutionary in a profession still largely operating with an apprenticeship model of training and unstructured assessment of juniors by their seniors (see below). Moreover, the pace of change is fast. By the time this report is published, all of the royal colleges are expected to have produced explicit training curricula setting out the skills doctors will need to achieve and how their competence should be measured, at least for the higher training grades.

The local structure of medical staffing in the 1990s

25. Such radical changes have impinged on almost all hospitals. Yet doctors retain many of their traditional working practices. Historically, hospital doctors worked in 'firms' – a consultant leading a team of 'his own' junior doctors of various grades. The firm had two main rationales:

- to ensure continuity of patient care by restricting an individual patient's contact to a small number of doctors. Providing 24-hour cover within a single firm requires doctors to work long hours in a single stretch. At one time junior doctors effectively lived at their hospitals for weeks at a time and emergency cover was provided from within each firm. Now, however, their hours of work are restricted and the pressure of work has increased. Firms now almost invariably comprise two or more consultants 'sharing' at least some of the junior staff, and doctors provide emergency cover to all patients in the specialty when they are on duty at night. In this sense continuity of patient care is already much reduced;

- to provide an apprenticeship style of medical training for junior doctors. The essence of apprenticeship training is close contact between a trainer and trainee. At one time juniors could follow the day-to-day work of their consultants around the hospital. Now, however, the different grades are often located in different settings (Box 1) and their commitments mean that the scope for apprenticeship-style training is much diminished.

26. Despite some broadening of firms and sharing of junior doctors, many consultants still practice as individuals rather than as part of a team and the roles of the junior grades and the culture of the medical hierarchy remain essentially the same. Doctors' working arrangements have not adapted fast enough to the rapidly changing environment in which they work. The next three chapters explore the implications of this for patient care and medical training.

Box 1
The roles of the different grades of doctors

Consultants predominantly work in outpatient clinics and operating theatres, with some formal ward rounds each week and informal contact with wards when required. They are also involved in a variety of non-clinical work, such as teaching, research and management and have ultimate legal responsibility for patients under their care.

Registrars and senior registrars, like consultants, work predominantly in outpatient clinics and operating theatres, but they tend to have more contact with wards. Like the consultants, much of their time is also taken up on correspondence, research and formal training activities, but not usually on management tasks.

Senior house officers (SHOs) spend most of their time on ward work and to a lesser extent in outpatient clinics and operating theatres. They provide most of the ward cover in specialties without a house officer.

House officers (HOs) are almost entirely ward-based.

Associate specialists are close to consultant status and tend to work in a way similar to consultants, although they are technically accountable to a consultant for all their patients.

Staff grade doctors may fit into the picture in many different ways, but tend to work on shifts and in specific clinical areas.

All grades can be involved in providing emergency cover. There are usually four separate rotas corresponding to the four main grades with associate specialist and staff grade doctors contributing to them if appropriate. The most junior grades are usually first on-call and are resident in the hospital when they are on duty. Consultants will be on-call in the hospital during the day and at home outside normal working hours. Occasionally, senior training grade doctors will also be on-call at home outside normal working hours.

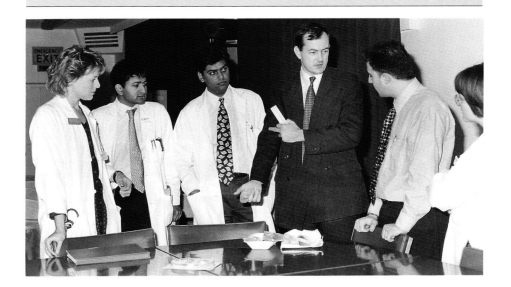

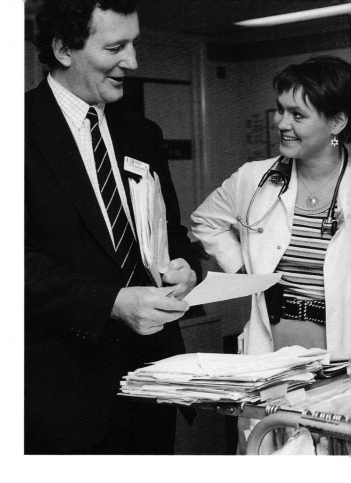

2 Skill Mix and Deployment

Many of doctors' working practices derive from long-standing customs and a culture of 'learning on the job'

The result is:

– hospitals differ in the allocation of tasks between doctors and other professions and the extent of supervision of junior doctors; and

– the number and mix of staff are more related to custom and practice than to the needs of either patient care or medical training.

Some doctors feel unsupported in their work because there is very little opportunity to work part-time and the working environment is sometimes poor.

A more systematic approach to skill mix and deployment is needed, with proper written job descriptions and clearer responsibilities and guidelines on who should do what. More flexibility is needed in the allocation of doctors' hours, the number of tiers in on-call rotas, the potential for shift working, the scope of emergency cover across the specialties and the nature of employment opportunities. Where necessary, facilities for doctors should be improved.

27. The primary role of NHS acute hospital trusts is to provide high quality patient care as efficiently and effectively as possible. They must also meet the requirements for training. Sometimes these objectives conflict. To achieve both objectives it is vital that the availability, grades and skills of doctors they employ are properly and explicitly matched to patients' needs and to medical training requirements, while maintaining safe levels of staffing which do not put patients at risk. A number of problems need to be overcome, many of which have their roots in long-standing working practices.

The problems

Lack of clarity of what doctors should do

28. The boundaries between the roles of doctors and those of the other professions involved in patient care are often not clear, and systems for allocating tasks between the different grades of doctors are lacking. This is particularly true for doctors in the most junior grade:

'In most of the PRHO [Pre-registration house officer] jobs, information about their timetables and the way consultants managed certain types of conditions, discharge arrangements etc. were acquired from notes left by the previous house officer, ward sisters and ward receptionists. SHOs and registrars were the key informants if they had worked with the firm previously, but PRHOs and SHOs often changed jobs on the same day'
(Ref. 10).

Over 40 per cent of junior doctors surveyed by the Audit Commission did not have job descriptions. Many of the doctors who did have them said they did not cover important aspects of their work (Exhibit 8).

Exhibit 8
Use of job descriptions for training grade doctors

Many doctors do not have job descriptions, and for those that do the job descriptions often do not cover important areas of their work.

Sample size: 386.

Source: Audit Commission.

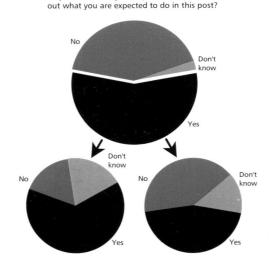

Have you ever been given a job description setting out what you are expected to do in this post?

No / Don't know / Yes

Did it set out the service component of the job?

Don't know / No / Yes

Did it set out the training and educational component of the job?

No / Don't know / Yes

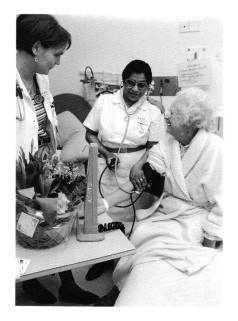

The result is

◆ hospitals differ in how tasks are divided between junior doctors and nurses or other professional groups. In many hospitals nurses and other professionals are now working in areas which were traditionally regarded as the province of doctors. These changes are the result mainly of attempts to reduce junior doctors' hours of work or of responses to difficulties encountered in recruiting doctors. They address only part of the skill mix question; the interface between junior doctors and other professions, e.g.:

– nurse practitioners in A&E departments, and sometimes in wards, who carry out basic duties like clerking patients (taking a patient's personal details and medical history) and insertion of intravenous cannulae;

– clinical nurse specialists, who work independently but according to guidelines agreed with doctors, have taken on some of the work previously done by doctors, principally in areas like intensive care, diabetes and care of the terminally ill;

– midwives who are carrying out the tasks of some junior doctors in obstetrics (Ref. 11);

– new categories of support workers like phlebotomists and ECG technicians; and

– non-medically trained surgeons' assistants who have been trained to do simple operations and procedures, notably in cardiac surgery. They work under direct supervision of a consultant who is responsible for their work. Their tasks may also include assisting the surgeon at operations and clerking patients;

◆ junior doctors do some tasks that do not require their specific skills. Relatively junior doctors are likely to do more of these tasks and all grades are more likely to do them at night than they are during the day (Exhibit 9).

Exhibit 9
'Inappropriate' tasks undertaken by training grade doctors

Relatively junior doctors do more of these tasks and all grades are more likely to do them at night.

Sample size: 206.

Methodology: Doctors at each of the study sites were asked which of six basic tasks, not specifically requiring medical training, they undertook 'frequently', 'occasionally' or 'never'. Their responses for each task were given a score of two, one and zero respectively. Thus a doctor undertaking all six 'inappropriate' tasks frequently would score a maximum of 12. Tasks included were: the pursuit of test results, the collection of equipment from wards, the setting up of intravenous infusions, the administering of intravenous drugs (excluding thrombolytic drugs), the taking of venous blood samples and recording of ECGs. The numbers are intended to show the differences between the grades and time of day.

Source: Audit Commission.

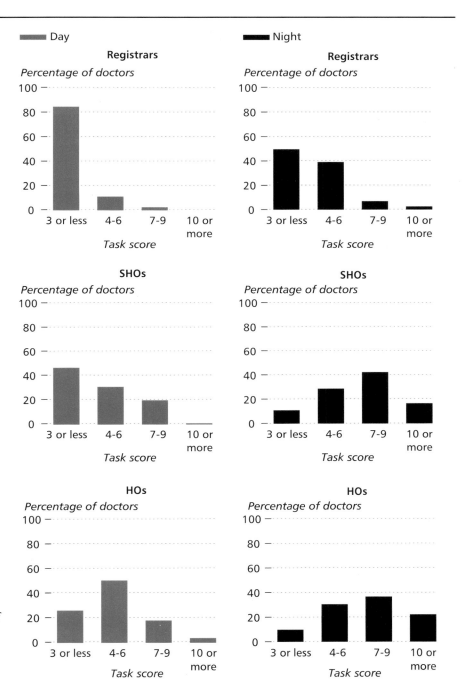

Insufficient supervision of junior doctors

29. All doctors below consultant rely on referring to their seniors if they need help. The success of this system rests on everyone knowing when they should seek help. But without some formal allocation of tasks and duties, the boundaries of individual action cannot be clear. This can become problematic when junior doctors think (rightly or wrongly) that a request for help may be viewed by their seniors as a sign of weakness or ignorance.

30. The most junior doctors are usually the first on the scene in emergencies and sometimes have too much responsibility given their level of training. Even in areas such as operating theatres and outpatient clinics, where consultants are generally thought to have much more involvement than in out-of-hours emergency work, supervision may be poor. Some variation between hospitals in the amount of operating SHOs do unsupervised is to be expected because of differences in the nature of the operations and their individual competence to carry them out, but not to the extent found by the Audit Commission. In some hospitals SHOs are undertaking most of their operations without a more senior doctor being present (Exhibit 10). So either they are being asked to operate alone beyond their competence or else they are being used only for operations they can already do and not having their competence extended. And SHOs run as many as 20 per cent of outpatient

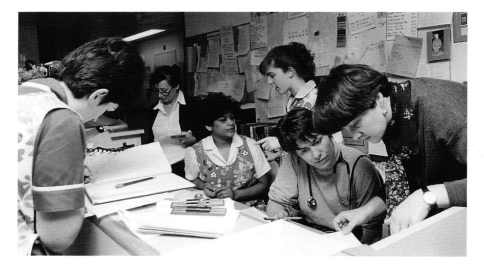

Exhibit 10
Percentage of operations where SHOs work alone or with a more junior doctor

In many hospitals SHOs are undertaking most of their operations without a senior being present.

Note: Vertical axes show hospital code number (each bar represents one hospital); horizontal axes show percentage of operations when SHOs were working alone or with an equal or more junior grade doctor.

Source: Audit Commission.

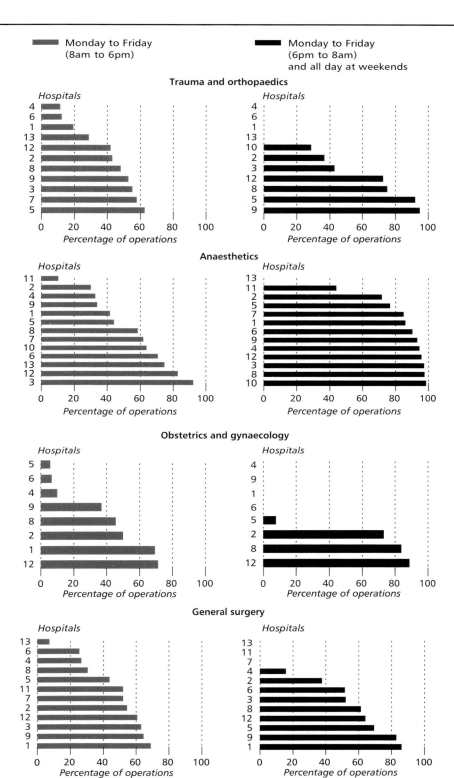

Exhibit 11
Outpatient clinics where SHOs were the most senior doctor on duty

SHOs run as many as 20 per cent of outpatient clinics in some hospitals.

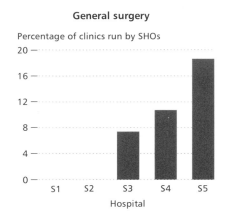

General surgery

Percentage of clinics run by SHOs

Hospital

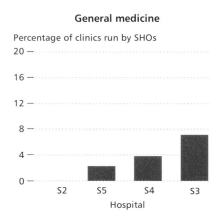

General medicine

Percentage of clinics run by SHOs

Hospital

Source: Audit Commission.

clinics in general medicine and general surgery in some hospitals (Exhibit 11). There is, incidentally, no suggestion that these practices reflect hospital policy – it is usually confined to one or two specialties.

31. It is often acceptable for training grade doctors to see patients on their own during outpatient clinics if they are properly supported before and afterwards. However, reported use of these indirect methods of supervision is not high and varies according to who is asked. For example, 47 per cent of consultants say that juniors present cases to them after clinics, but only 20 per cent of juniors concur with this assessment (Exhibit 12). If senior doctors are reviewing case notes and GPs' letters prepared by juniors without telling them, then communication between them is poor and there is a lack of feedback.

32. Inadequate supervision of junior doctors has implications for their career progression as well as for patient care. There is little hard information on which to base an assessment of career prospects. In common with many other professions, career progression for doctors is based largely on subjective assessment of their competence and potential, but the circumstances of hospital medicine make it difficult to build up the necessary degree of knowledge on which to base such assessments. Junior doctors tend to move frequently between hospitals and to some extent also between specialties, and the large size of many hospitals and differences in the nature of work of consultants and juniors limit contact between them. In these circumstances there is a risk that consultants will take the confidence of a junior to carry out specific tasks as a proxy for their ability (Ref. 10). Junior doctors' confidence in performing cardio-pulmonary resuscitation, for example, relates more to the number they have attended than to any objective assessment of their skills (Ref. 12).

Exhibit 12
Perceptions of the way juniors are supervised when they see new outpatients

Consultants and junior doctors differ markedly in their perception of supervision.

	% of consultants answering yes	% of juniors answering yes
Case notes reviewed by a more senior doctor before clinic	57	29
Case notes reviewed by a senior doctor after clinic	18	10
Junior accompanied by senior	29	7
Junior presents case to senior after clinic	47	20
Senior reviews letters to be sent to GPs	18	10
SAMPLE SIZE	119	198

Source: Audit Commission.

Demand is seldom allocated or managed

33. Traditionally individual patients are referred personally to consultants by GPs or by other consultants. The relative size of consultants' caseloads (and therefore of doctors working with them) is affected by the number of referrals they receive. This can result in significant differences in workload between consultants, making it more difficult to deploy doctors of all grades to meet demand efficiently (see Chapter 3).

34. In most hospitals schedules for outpatient and operating theatre sessions have built up incrementally over many years, and the overall implications for medical staffing have not been reviewed. There is evidence that a third of general surgical and orthopaedic operations carried out as emergencies at night could be delayed until the next day (Ref. 13) if operating theatre capacity were available. Moreover, the confidential national enquiry into perioperative deaths has shown that better outcomes are likely if this is done (Ref. 14). Yet few hospitals have rationalised the generally piecemeal approach to the use of operating theatres for emergencies, for example, by grouping them into daily scheduled sessions.

Workload and staff availability are poorly matched

35. Most hospitals operate with only two levels of medical staffing: weekday daytime hours (generally 9 a.m. to 5 p.m.) and on-call duties at all other times. But the peaks in emergency referrals tend to occur in the late morning and early evening. This pattern suggests that there may be too many doctors on duty during parts of the day, too few in the evening and too many again at night, particularly in those specialties with a high proportion of emergency work such as general medicine and care of the elderly. Moreover, in many cases the intensity of non-emergency ward work and the demands of training vary considerably across the working day.

36. On-call rotas which determine the out-of-hours cover will be inefficient and contribute to the long hours worked by many junior doctors if they

Exhibit 13
Number of tiers in on-call rotas

Most hospitals had 'standard' three- or four-tier rotas, depending on the specialty.

Includes general medicine, general surgery and obstetrics and gynaecology. The 'standard' rota is one of four tiers (consultant, senior registrar/registrar, SHO and HO) in general medicine and surgery and three tiers in obstetrics and gynaecology (house officers do not work in this specialty). Usually one doctor is on duty at each level, although sometimes in very large hospitals more than one doctor may be on duty at each level.

Source: Ref. 15 and Audit Commission.

Dowie survey 1987
28 rotas in 11 hospitals (including two teaching hospitals)

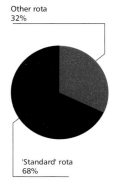

Other rota
32%

'Standard' rota
68%

Audit Commission study sites 1993
19 rotas in 7 hospitals (including one teaching hospital)

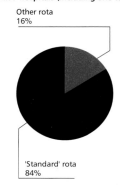

Other rota
16%

'Standard' rota
84%

include more tiers of doctors than are necessary for the demands of the service and training. In many hospitals rotas are based on three tiers (four tiers where house officers are included) of medical staff working in a single specialty (Exhibit 13). If the workload is sufficient to justify this number of doctors and the skill mix is appropriate to the nature of the work, there is no problem. But in many cases, as the uniformity of the rotas suggests, it is custom and practice rather than the nature of the work or the risk of emergency 'peaks', which determine the number of tiers in the rota.

Many doctors feel unsupported in their work

37. Many women, and increasingly men, face personal and family commitments which make it difficult for them to pursue a medical career under current conditions of employment. Although the percentage of women doctors has increased over the years, and over 50 per cent of those now entering medicine are women (Ref. 16), the more senior posts remain predominantly filled by men (Exhibit 14). The fact that women are more likely to move into areas of medicine outside hospital or leave medicine altogether is almost certainly an indication of the problems they face in pursuing a hospital career (Ref. 2). This is a serious problem for both individual trusts and the NHS as a whole. It is inefficient and wasteful to train any group of staff to such high levels and then fail to make maximum use of their potential. The main underlying problems that need urgent attention are:

◆ **Unnecessarily onerous on-call requirements.** This issue was raised spontaneously by 40 per cent of women respondents and nearly a third of men in a recent major survey of doctors' careers and was by far the single most important factor seen by them to impose a constraint on their careers (Ref. 16).

◆ **Poor career advice**, going back as far as medical school. At the time they have to make crucial decisions about their future careers, few women are aware of the difficulties they will face in trying to combine a medical career with having children. Eighty-five per cent of UK-qualified doctors who move into the staff grade are women. About half of these had not received career advice in the 12 months prior to taking up the post and many still

24

Exhibit 14
The representation of women in the medical workforce in England and Wales, 1973-1992

Although the number of women doctors has increased as a percentage of all doctors over the years, the imbalance between the grades has remained.

Source: Department of Health, Health and Personal Social Services Statistics.

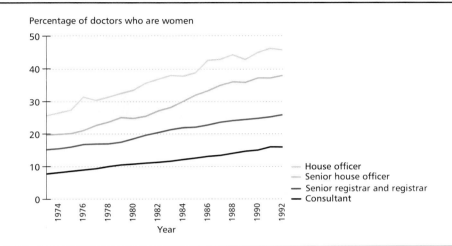

Percentage of doctors who are women

House officer
Senior house officer
Senior registrar and registrar
Consultant

Year

aspire to consultant status even though the staff grade is intended as a final career grade (Ref.17).

◆ **The lack of suitable part-time career posts.** Most women doctors and many male doctors think that there is a need for more part-time career posts (Ref. 16), while acknowledging that part-time work is regarded as being lower status than full-time.

38. There are also problems associated with inflexible training structures and processes which tend to have a greater impact on women than men (see Chapter 4, page 54).

39. Consultants and junior doctors often justifiably complain of poor facilities. Apart from parking which is almost invariably a problem for staff and patients, junior doctors highlight the doctors' mess (common room or staff room), on-call sleeping accommodation and catering as the main areas where facilities are poor (Exhibit 15). The particular importance of good facilities for junior doctors' unsocial hours is recognised in the *New Deal*.

Exhibit 15
Facilities identified by training grade doctors as being poor

Parking, the doctors' mess and the on-call accommodation are areas regarded by many doctors as being poor.

Source: Audit Commission.

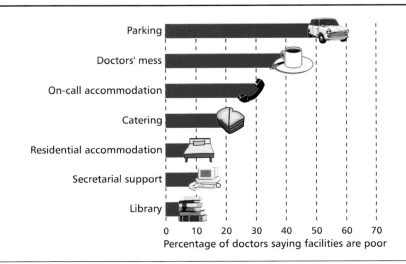

Parking
Doctors' mess
On-call accommodation
Catering
Residential accommodation
Secretarial support
Library

Percentage of doctors saying facilities are poor

Overcoming the problems

40. Tackling these problems will not be easy. Long-standing, sometimes deeply ingrained practices will need to change. There are encouraging signs, however, that some doctors both understand the need for change and are prepared to meet the challenge (page 30).

Define doctors' roles in relation to other professions

41. The new professional roles being developed in many trusts and aimed at reducing junior doctors' hours of work (page 18), can bring considerable benefits (Box 2). But the benefits could be much greater if they are part of a broader policy to change skill mix. It is not just a matter of considering the role of junior doctors. All grades, including consultants, should be considered part of such a policy.

42. The patient-focused care approach, for example, being adopted in some hospitals, combines definition of roles with a wider reorganisation of care. Most of the services commonly needed by patients in a particular department can be grouped into small, self-contained physical units. Staff, including doctors, are allocated to these units. Patient care is improved because the services needed by patients are in closer proximity and they can be coordinated more effectively and used more efficiently. Doctors benefit because their work is more concentrated in one location rather than spread widely across the hospital. Professional boundaries can be broken down, allowing staff to be used more flexibly to meet patient needs. The approach provides an opportunity to develop guidelines on the roles of each of the professions because all staff working in these units work more closely together.

43. Such fundamental changes have wide implications for training in the different professions. The Government, together with the bodies responsible for medical and nursing training, should monitor these changes. They need to ensure that, where appropriate, training adapts to demand for new combinations of knowledge and skills.

Box 2
New professional roles supporting doctors

1. Support Worker Scheme, Northern General Hospital, Sheffield

Duties include:

- taking blood;
- putting up drips;
- recording ECGs; and
- clerical work.

Benefits:

- routine tasks removed from doctors' duties;
- doctor contact with patients increased from 14 per cent to 18 per cent of time on duty;
- doctors hours of work reduced because they are able to have half a day off each week; and
- routine tasks better organised with
  - easier to arrange tests and investigations,
  - tasks performed sooner,
  - IV drugs no longer missed because of lack of a cannula and
  - request forms more legible with fewer mistakes. *Source: Audit Commission.*

2. Cardiac Surgeon's Assistant, Oxford Heart Centre, John Radcliffe Hospital

Duties include:

- assisting in theatre including removal of saphenous veins from the legs;
- admitting patients to ward, e.g.
  - filling forms,
  - ordering pre-operative tests and X-rays,
  - carrying out phlebotomies and line insertion;
- post-operative care, e.g.
  - assessment of wound care in clinic,
  - giving discharge advice; and
- specialist services, e.g.
  - procuring homografts,
  - operating the intra-aortic balloon pump and
  - performing exercise stress tests.

Benefits:

- specialist assistance on wards and in theatre which junior doctors are unable to provide;
- junior doctors relieved of long periods spent in operating theatre with little training benefit;
- provides continuity in the department; and
- ability to teach junior doctors basic surgical skills and to train other hospital staff in resuscitation techniques *Source: Ref. 18.*

Clarify the allocation of tasks and supervision

44. All doctors should have a job description setting out the service and training components of their work. Tasks should be allocated to the most appropriate profession and grade with the required level of quality and competence. General principles and guidelines should be developed to inform junior doctors what level of supervision they should receive and when they should seek advice. Such guidelines should help to ensure that consultants are more aware of their supervisory responsibilities and should result in greater consistency of practice. More specific guidelines are also needed dealing with the management of the most common conditions, particularly where more than one department is involved (e.g. acute upper gastro-intestinal bleeding and deliberate self-harm). Responsibilities can often be made much clearer simply by formalising existing procedures.

45. When these principles are applied, the boundaries of action for the main grades should become clearer (Exhibit 16). However, much depends on the way in which 'competence' is assessed. The royal colleges are moving towards clearer specification of the tasks and procedures that doctors should be capable of performing at each stage in their training, but it will be some years before these will take effect (see Chapter 4). In the meantime trusts will have to rely on their own assessment methods.

46. Junior doctors should have access to a consultant at all times and in all settings (operating theatres, outpatient clinics and wards) in the absence of an individual patient's named consultant. One consultant for the specialty should be designated to be available for juniors to contact and should be empowered to take decisions about the care of individual patients. This is important to avoid delays which may be detrimental to patient care. But to work effectively it requires teamwork between consultants and agreements on basic clinical approaches.

47. House officers should always be on duty with another more senior doctor. Some reduction in their hours of work should be possible in those instances where they are on duty purely for training purposes and not to provide service cover. They should not need to be on duty 24 hours a day for training purposes and the evidence on the amount of training they receive suggests that they will not lose out if the hours are reduced (Ref. 10).

Manage demand

48. Changes can be made to the way in which patients are allocated to individual consultants:

◆ Some specialties are now agreeing with local GPs referral systems for outpatients and elective inpatients, which do not specify an individual consultant and allow the specialty to allocate the patient to a consultant according to workload and other factors. This practice offers much more flexibility in staffing the service, but does not rule out a personal referral where doctors or patients want it.

Exhibit 16
Example of the allocation of tasks between consultants and trainees

The boundaries of action for all grades should be much clearer.

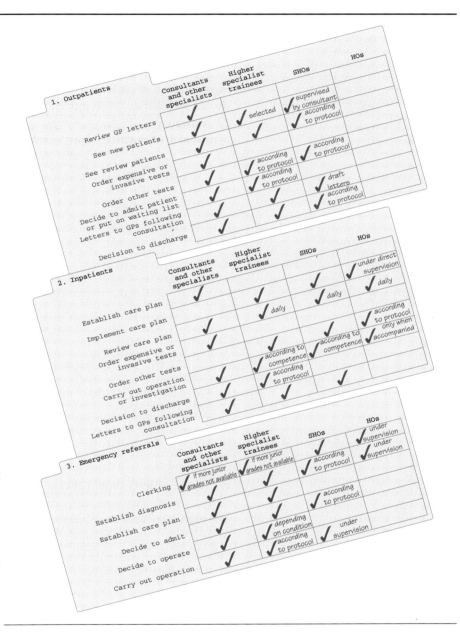

Note: The roles are set out according to the new grade definitions recommended in the Calman Report (Ref.9) and are largely based on existing guidance and established good practice: e.g. General Medical Council, *Recommendations on General Clinical Training* (1992) and *Recommendations on the Training of Specialists* (1987); Royal College of Physicians, *General Professional Training: A Guide for Trainees and Trainers* (1993); The Surgical Royal Colleges of Great Britain and Ireland, *Guidelines for Basic Surgical Training* (1994). They are, however, intended only as an example of what is needed locally, not as a blueprint.

Source: Audit Commission.

- ◆ Patients admitted as emergencies can also be distributed between consultants more evenly. Some hospitals, for example, allocate each consultant a ward or block of beds. Each new emergency patient is admitted under whichever consultant is on duty for the specialty, and transferred to the consultant who 'owns' that bed when they are next on duty in the hospital. This arrangement evens out the emergency workload, but again requires team-work between consultants including agreements on shared responsibilities and consistency on basic approaches to patient care.

49. Trusts should review operating theatre and outpatient clinic timetables with consultants so as to achieve a more efficient allocation of sessions and doctors. And they should consider introducing emergency operating sessions into theatre schedules during the daytime or evening to avoid unnecessary operations at night.

Deploy doctors according to the demand

50. The regional teams of doctors and managers responsible for implementing the *New Deal* (page 13) are actively considering new approaches to deployment to reduce hours of work. In Anglia and Oxford region, for example, they have suggested a new regime which includes (Ref. 19):

- more senior doctors on duty to meet the relatively high level of emergency referrals in the late morning and evening, with a compensating reduction in the level of cover after midnight. This is also to help avoid unnecessary and often distressing long waits experienced by some patients at the end of the day;

- arranging schedules that allow consultants to see their emergency patients earlier so that they can be quickly assessed and treated;

- minimising emergency call-out of junior doctors at night by:

  - encouraging them to do a final (short) ward round at the end of the day to anticipate likely calls over night;

  - clarifying with nurses the circumstances for which a doctor should be called out (e.g. to confirm all deaths or only unexpected ones); and

- establishing a dedicated area for emergency referrals and patients likely to develop complications overnight so that the area can be efficiently staffed by doctors working a shift system.

There may also be scope for organising junior doctors' hours more flexibly during the normal working day to take account of the fluctuations in service and training demands.

Greater use of shifts

51. The organisation of the on-call emergency cover should be determined by the nature of demand. Where possible, emergency cover should be provided using shift and partial-shift systems. They are a more effective use of doctors' time and many junior doctors prefer them. Two thirds of recently qualified doctors say they have experienced shifts or partial shifts (mainly when working in accident and emergency departments) and two thirds of the same sample said they prefer them (Ref. 16). Compared to rota systems, shifts:

- mean that doctors on duty are less tired than they would be on a rota system; they work fewer hours and are less likely to have had their sleep interrupted;

'The organisation of the on-call emergency cover should be determined by the nature of demand'

◆ give a precise specification of the number of hours to be worked; and

◆ offer opportunity for better training as the number and grades of doctors actually working 'out-of-hours' is more predictable, whereas with a rota system it depends on who is called out. The quality and quantity of training should also improve if doctors are less tired.

But shift and partial-shift systems require more doctors to operate them than conventional on-call rotas and so can only be considered where the demand is sufficient. There must also be sufficient spare capacity to cope with emergency peaks, perhaps through joint arrangements with other specialties. Nevertheless, it is likely to be difficult, if not impossible, to meet the requirements of the *New Deal* for shorter hours of work without changes such as these.

52. Doctors sometimes object to shifts, principally because they see them as a threat to the continuity of patient care (Ref. 20), but shifts might provide greater continuity of care if the same doctor is on duty at the same time each day. In any case, rotas often do not provide continuity either (see page 14). No system will ensure continuity unless it includes formal rules about handover, including between 30 and 60 minutes protected time for that purpose. Handover should include other professional staff involved in patient care. Effective handover arrangements can also become a valuable part of training.

Reduce the number of tiers in on-call rotas

53. If the quantity of work is not sufficient to justify the number of tiers in a rota providing on-call cover, consideration should be given to reducing the number of tiers as long as the scope of the work is within the competence of the doctors involved and they have clear rules about when to seek advice from a senior. This will necessitate increased flexibility about who does what. Consultants will sometimes need to carry out work that could be done by registrars, but this extra work will be offset as the number of consultants increases. Even in cases where the quantity of work is sufficient to justify the number of doctors on duty, it may be more appropriate to deploy more doctors at the same grade rather than having three or four tiers in the rota.

Combine specialties for emergency cover

54. Increasing specialisation over recent years has meant that the basic unit of medical staffing – the specialty – has become smaller and smaller. Independent emergency rotas are no longer viable in many of the smaller specialties. The answer is to share emergency cover with other specialties, depending on the competence of the doctors involved. Whilst it would obviously be unwise to combine, say, obstetrics with cardiology at anything other than SHO level (and even that is questionable), there is greater opportunity for joint working within the main medical specialties or surgical specialties as happens in many other countries.

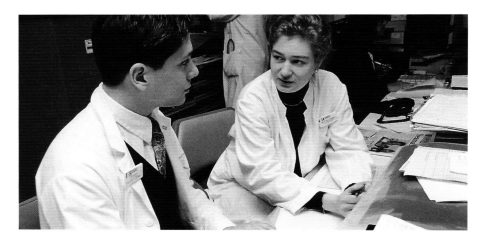

Provide better employment opportunities and support

55. Providing posts and career paths which are equally accessible to the growing number of doctors with family commitments is essential for the efficient running of the NHS as well as the career prospects of the individuals involved. Many of the recommendations already made will go some way to reducing the long hours of work which are the major barrier.

56. Proper career advice is essential at medical school and right through a doctor's hospital career. Postgraduate deans who are responsible for doctors in the training grades should encourage trusts to provide them with more career advice. Existing national and local advice schemes aimed specifically at women doctors could be more widely publicised, for example, the Women in Surgical Training (WIST) support group set up by the Royal College of Surgeons.

57. But better career advice is not a substitute for more accessible posts. More part-time posts are needed in all the career grades and training grades (page 59). This could be achieved by more job sharing and by the use of a greater variety of posts covering different types of work. Specialties with high proportions of elective patients are most suitable for part-time work but, even in specialties with heavy emergency workloads, shifts and rotas can be organised to accommodate part-time work. The perception of many doctors that part-time work has a relatively low status is partly a function of its rarity for both the career and training grades. It should become more acceptable as it becomes more widespread.

58. The Audit Commission will be examining facilities in the local audits of medical staffing. This will be coordinated with similar inspections being carried out by postgraduate deans and regional *New Deal* task-forces. Postgraduate deans have a mechanism for persuading trusts to improve facilities, where necessary, through the contract for medical training. Trusts should in any case seek to ensure that facilities reach the standard set out in the *New Deal* guidelines (Ref. 6). Facilities are a major part of the working environment and are important in doctors' job satisfaction. Through this they may also have an effect on patient care.

Conclusion

59. The Audit Commission's recommendations on skill mix and deployment are primarily about making:

◆ working practices more formal so that competence and responsibility are clear; and

◆ criteria for deployment more explicit so that staff are allocated efficiently to meet the demands of patient care and training.

The recommendations need to be implemented in a coordinated and consistent way as part of a medical staffing plan that covers day-to-day staffing matters as well as setting out the major changes needed (Exhibit 17). Such a plan should, for example, include arrangements for doctors' absences which are a source of potential disruption. All absences should be planned as far as possible in advance. Prospective cover should be built into the timetables and staffing levels, anticipating both the complexity and quantity of work likely to be done. Responsibilities for drawing up and implementing the staff plan fall naturally to the medical and clinical directors in a trust. The task must also be coordinated with responsibilities for meeting training needs which are discussed in Chapter 4. Management arrangements for meeting both service and training needs are discussed in Chapter 5.

Exhibit 17
A medical staffing plan

Trusts need a plan that covers both day-to-day staffing matters and plans for major changes.

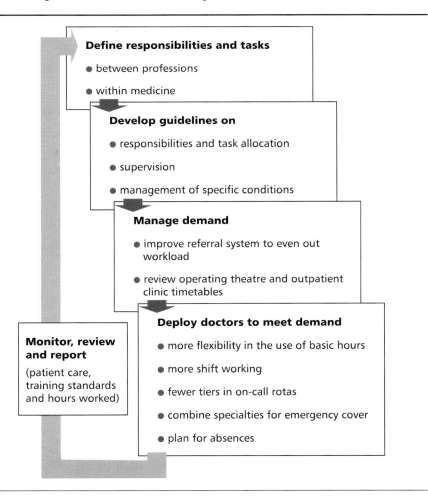

Source: Audit Commission.

33

34

60. The consequences of changing the number of doctors employed, their skill mix and their deployment are complex. In some cases, where additional consultants or staff grade doctors are needed to do some of the work previously carried out by training grades, extra expenditure will be necessary. This could, in part, be offset by implementing some of the recommendations in this chapter, such as matching hours of work and the number of tiers in rotas, more closely to service and training needs.

Recommendations on skill mix and deployment

Trusts

1 Trusts should clarify the roles of doctors and other professions by:

- ensuring that all doctors have job descriptions setting out the service and training content of their work;
- developing clear written guidelines about the allocation of tasks between doctors and other professions and between the different grades of doctors;
- ensuring that tasks are efficiently matched to the competence of the doctors involved.

2 Policies should be developed by trusts **in cooperation with postgraduate deans** on the nature and extent of supervision of junior doctors. Juniors must know when to seek help and seniors must be aware of their responsibilities.

3 Junior doctors should at all times have access to a consultant who has the power to make decisions about the care of individual patients in the absence of a patient's named consultant.

4 Trusts should manage demand more effectively and encourage consultants to share the workload more evenly. Where possible, patients awaiting emergency operations should be grouped into scheduled sessions.

5 Doctors should be deployed more efficiently to meet both service and training needs:

- junior doctors, basic working hours should be allocated more flexibly across the day;
- shift and partial-shift systems should be encouraged because they offer advantages to both patients and doctors;
- protected time for handover between shifts and rotas is needed to ensure continuity of patient care;
- the number of tiers of staff providing emergency cover should be reduced if the demand is not sufficient for the current number; and
- where appropriate, specialties should also be combined to provide emergency cover.

6 Trusts must develop policies and posts **in cooperation with postgraduate deans and the royal colleges** to take account of the special needs of doctors with family commitments.

7   Trusts should develop a medical staffing plan to implement the recommended changes in a coherent framework. This should include details about day-to-day working arrangements at specialty level as well as the more strategic issues at hospital level.

Other bodies

8   The **Government, together with the bodies responsible for medical and nursing training,** should monitor the changing roles of the different professions involved in health care and ensure that training adapts to reflect them.

9   Better career advice is essential and **postgraduate deans and the royal colleges** should publicise the schemes they already have in place and develop new ones.

10   **Postgraduate deans, regional *New Deal* taskforces and trusts themselves** should ensure that doctors' working conditions, especially the on-call facilities are of a sufficiently high standard.

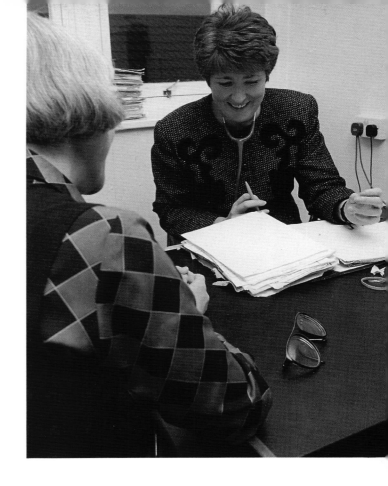

3 The Contribution of Consultants

Many consultants do not have job plans and, for those that do, they are often out of date.

The number of outpatient and operating theatre sessions consultants attend varies widely even within individual specialties and hospitals.

The number of patients consultants operate on or see in clinics, after allowing for differences in case complexity, is determined more by the number of sessions they attend than by the speed of their work.

Surgeons and anaesthetists doing relatively large amounts of private practice do less NHS work than their colleagues.

Job plans should be completed for all consultants and they should specify exactly what is expected of each consultant. The reasons for consultants having less than seven fixed commitments should be made clear. Attendance of consultants at fixed commitments (e.g. outpatient clinics and operating theatre sessions) should be monitored on a sample basis. Trusts also have a duty to ask consultants to state the extent of their private practice. Job plans should be regularly reviewed.

61. Consultants play a pivotal role in meeting both service and training needs. They determine the quality and quantity of most medical care and treatment that individual patients receive and are legally responsible for its delivery, whether or not they are personally involved. Their role in directing and managing other doctors has been discussed in the previous chapter and will be taken up further in Chapters 4 and 5. This chapter is concerned with their personal contribution to meeting service needs, and focuses on the mechanisms by which consultants implement the service objectives and standards set by trusts and on the nature of consultants' individual inputs. These are major components of ensuring value for money and high quality care.

62. Consultants have considerable autonomy to determine their work patterns. Prior to the formation of the NHS many consultants held honorary unpaid appointments at voluntary public hospitals and had considerable freedom of action. At that time they derived much of their income from private medical practice and teaching fees. When the NHS was formed they became salaried staff, but much of the freedom they had enjoyed in voluntary hospitals continued in custom and practice. In particular, they retained the right to undertake private practice.

63. There is little doubt that the majority of consultants, like most professionals, work long hours (Ref. 21) and that their non-clinical duties (such as management duties, clinical audit, teaching and other responsibilities) have increased in recent years (Ref. 22). They have also had to face change in medical practice and in the NHS, unprecedented in both its pace and extent. So there is all the more reason for trust managers and doctors alike to reassure themselves that the work that consultants do is in line with their trust's commitments to patient care and medical training and that the burden of work is fairly shared.

The problems

Inadequate use of job plans

64. In 1991 district health authorities (DHAs) and trusts were given greater control over consultants' contracts and the contracts were expected to contain job plans covering the individual consultant's responsibilities and programme of work. The rules state clearly (Ref. 23) that every consultant should have agreed a job plan with the chief executive or other senior manager of the trust, which states his or her fixed commitments in detail. These are commitments such as outpatient clinics and operating theatre sessions which:

'...a consultant must fulfil, except by agreement with local management or in an emergency, because otherwise the use of other health service resources would be adversely affected' (Ref. 24).

In some hospitals, however, job plans do not exist and in many they do not contain all the required information or are out of date. In a small sample of six hospitals only three were able to produce a complete set of them (Exhibit 18). The full extent of this problem will be investigated in the local audits.

65. Both whole-time and maximum-part-time consultants are effectively employed for ten 'notional half days' (NHDs), or periods of 3.5 hours. The difference between the two types of contracts relates to the right to undertake private practice (see page 44). The national guidelines on job plans state that:

'…for a consultant on a whole-time or maximum-part-time contract, between five and seven notional half days, depending on the specialty, should normally be allocated to fixed commitments…' (Ref. 24).

The guidance does not indicate where particular specialties should lie within the range of five to seven. The position on the range should relate mainly to on-call duties according to some of the guidance on consultant's contracts produced by the royal colleges (Ref. 25). Consultants with relatively onerous on-call duties (e.g. long hours or with no higher trainees to support them) might be expected to do fewer fixed commitments.

Exhibit 18
Existence of consultants' job plans

Only three out of six hospitals surveyed had a complete set of job plans available.

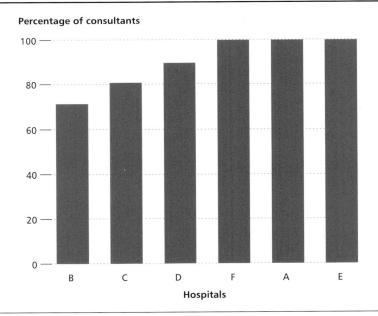

Percentage of consultants

Source: Audit Commission.

66. Examination of the job plans of 60 whole-time and maximum-part-time consultants – excluding those of doctors with significant non-clinical roles such as medical directors, clinical directors and clinical tutors – shows wide variation in the level of fixed commitments, which does not appear to be explained by on-call duties (Exhibit 19). Some consultants have more than seven fixed commitments (NHDs), which further accentuates the variation.

67. Irrespective of the number of fixed commitments in a consultant's job plan it is important to ensure that they are being fulfilled and very few trusts monitor this even on a sample basis. Surveys of consultants' activity in both operating theatres and outpatient clinics were undertaken over a six-week period and verified by local auditors to ascertain consultants' attendance rates against those stated in job plans and departmental timetables. Fifty-four per cent of consultants attended all their fixed commitments and a further 14 per cent attended between 90 and 99 per cent of these sessions during the sample period. These results exclude sessions missed due to sick leave, annual leave and study leave, and sessions which were cancelled for reasons outside a consultant's control (Exhibit 20).

Variation in consultants' workloads

68. After adjusting for case complexity, it is the number of fixed commitments attended rather than a consultant's speed of work which has the major effect on his or her quantity of work. But it is difficult to assess how much consultants do from routinely available NHS data both because such data generally counts patients for whom a consultant is nominally responsible, irrespective of which doctors actually carry out the work, and because it currently takes little or no account of differences in the complexity of the work. The Audit Commission has carried out its own surveys which overcome these problems as far as possible, covering both surgical and medical disciplines.

Exhibit 19
The relationship between the number of fixed commitments and on-call duties

The variation in the number of fixed commitments cannot be explained by a consultant's on-call duties.

Note: Fixed commitments include operating theatre sessions, outpatient and special procedure clinics (such as endoscopy) and ward rounds.

Sample size: 60 consultants (some points represent more than one observation).

Source: Audit Commission.

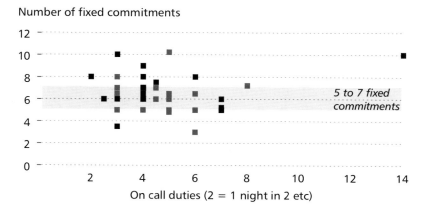

Number of fixed commitments

On call duties (2 = 1 night in 2 etc)

5 to 7 fixed commitments

■ General surgery, trauma and orthopaedics, urology, obstetrics & gynaecology
■ General medicine, care of the elderly

Exhibit 20
Consultants' attendance at fixed commitments

Sixty-eight per cent of consultants attended at least ninety per cent of all their fixed commitments.

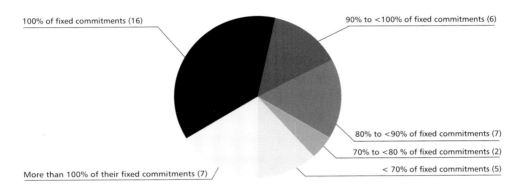

100% of fixed commitments (16)

90% to <100% of fixed commitments (6)

80% to <90% of fixed commitments (7)

70% to <80 % of fixed commitments (2)

< 70% of fixed commitments (5)

More than 100% of their fixed commitments (7)

Number of consultants (shown in brackets) attending.

Sample size: 43.

Fixed commitments in this case include operating theatre and outpatient sessions only. They were determined from job plans – where available – and clinic and operating theatre timetables. Sessions where a consultant was on annual leave, sick leave or study leave or where a clinic or operating list was cancelled for reasons outside a consultant's control are excluded. Some consultants do more than 100 per cent of sessions because they are providing cover for their colleagues' absences or have arranged additional sessions during the study period.

Source: Audit Commission.

Surgery

69. Lists of all operations carried out over a three-month period (April-June 1993) were obtained from ten hospitals spread throughout England and Wales. A detailed analysis of the work of 106 consultant surgeons in five specialties was carried out. The operations were standardised for differences in case complexity using the method explained in Appendix 4. The results show that some consultants do considerably more work than others, but primarily because they operate for more hours and to a lesser extent because they work faster[1]. And they operate for more hours mainly because they attend more sessions rather than because they operate over a longer period within each session (Exhibit 21, overleaf, and Appendix 4). In outpatient work the number

[1] That is not to say that some surgeons do not work faster than others. The results show an approximately two-fold variation in speed of operating. The point is that this variation is not a good predictor of their total weekly output.

of sessions attended dominates the quantity of output as it does for operating theatres (Appendix 6).

Medicine

70. Similarly, data on general physicians' work in outpatient clinics shows that the number of patients they see each week is related both to the number of clinics they attend and to the number of patients seen per hour (a measure which reflects both the speed of work of a consultant and the complexity of the cases – Exhibit 22).

Exhibit 21
The work of individual consultants in operating theatres – general surgery

The number of sessions attended each week is the main factor explaining differences in workload.

Sample size: 29.

Note: The methodology is explained in Appendix 4. Each bar represents one consultant. They are consistently ordered in each graph – based on case-mix-adjusted weekly output. Actual time 'at the table' is the time spent operating, ignoring the gaps between operations. The data are for daytime sessions defined as 8 a.m. to 1.30 p.m. and 1.30 p.m. to 6 p.m.

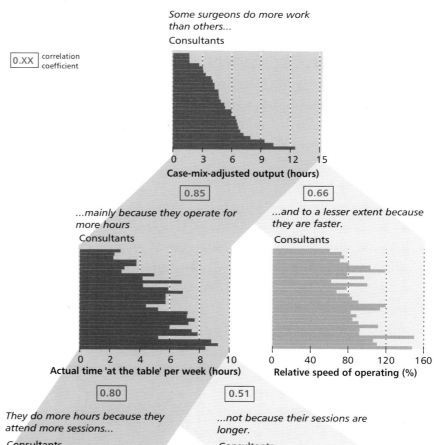

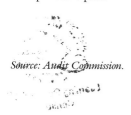

Source: Audit Commission.

71. One of the main reasons for the variation in consultants' contributions in both surgery and medicine is the personal referral system for GPs reported in the previous chapter (see page 23). The relatively low attendance of some consultants at operating theatre sessions and outpatient clinics may also be explained by factors beyond their control such as shortages of theatre and clinic capacity or a trust's restrictions on elective work. However, factors such as these are unlikely to explain the big differences observed within a single specialty and hospital. The effect of private practice on NHS work is another possible reason for variation in individuals' contributions.

Exhibit 22
The work of individual consultants in outpatient clinics – general medicine

The number of clinics attended per week is a major factor explaining differences in workloads.

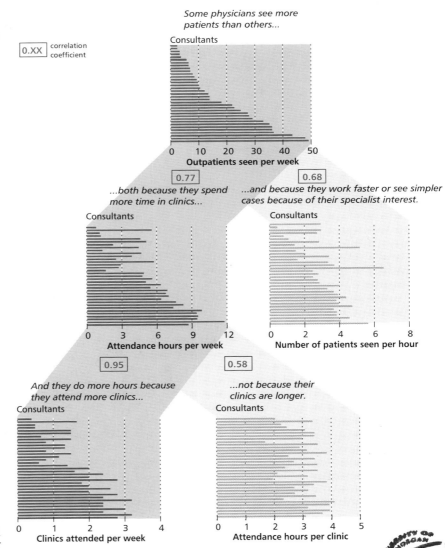

Sample size: 35 consultants.

Note: The methodology is explained in the text and in Appendix 6. Each bar represents one consultant. They are consistently ordered in each graph – based on outpatients seen per week.

Source: Audit Commission.

' ...the 25 per cent of consultants who do the most private work carry out less NHS work than their colleagues'

Private practice

72. The national terms and conditions of service for hospital medical staff allow all doctors to undertake private practice. For junior staff this must be limited to times when they are not contracted to work for the NHS, but for consultants there is no restriction on when it can take place. Such guidance as does exist is not very specific. Consultants on whole-time or maximum-part-time contracts are told that they should: *'...devote substantially the whole of their professional time to the NHS'* (Ref. 23). Consultants on whole-time NHS contracts must not, however, receive payments from private practice work in excess of the equivalent of ten per cent of their gross NHS salary. Consultants on maximum-part-time contracts forgo this restriction in exchange for a nine per cent reduction in their NHS salary. Over recent years the amount of private practice has been growing and consultants have seen faster growth in their private practice earnings than their NHS salaries (consultants' total earnings – NHS and private sector combined – grew by about ten per cent per year between 1980 and 1992 compared to growth of eight per cent per year in NHS pay alone over the same period – Ref. 26).

73. In order to test whether the quantity of consultants' NHS work is related to the amount of their private work, the Audit Commission obtained the cooperation of a number of private health insurers to provide a statistically reliable sample of private work which could be matched with its sample of NHS work containing 227 consultants (141 surgeons and 86 anaesthetists) from the ten hospitals surveyed (see page 41 and Appendices 4 and 5). The work of these individuals in the private sector was obtained for the same three-month period and adjusted for differences in complexity of cases in the same way as for their NHS work. For the majority of consultants there was no relationship between the amount of work performed in the private sector and the amount they carried out in the NHS, but the results did show that the 25 per cent of consultants who do the most private work carry out less NHS work than their colleagues; a result which was statistically significant (Appendix 5). If anything, the results are likely to be an underestimate of the trade-off between NHS and private work. For those so inclined, it is easier and less 'visible' to find the time for private practice by cutting back on aspects of NHS responsibilities other than operating sessions. However, further work should be carried out to build on these important preliminary findings.

Overcoming the problems

Better use of job plans

74. Job plans spelling out consultants' commitments should be a major part of contracts and job descriptions, whether consultants are employed under national terms and conditions of service or on local trust terms. They should be comprehensive, consistent, monitored and regularly reviewed (Exhibit 23).

Comprehensive

75. Job plans should be completed for all consultants and should specify all the responsibilities and duties expected of a consultant in addition to clinical work, including those for management, service development, teaching and research.

Consistent

76. NHS trusts should draw up guidelines for completing job plans, agreed with their consultants. These agreements might include, for example, the number of notional half days that are given in lieu of specific on-call commitments (taking account of the likelihood of actually being called and the degree of junior doctor support), and the administrative and other duties which consultants have in common.

77. The factors taken into account in arriving at the number of fixed commitments and the overall structure of the job plan should be explicit (i.e. on-call commitments, numbers of junior doctors for whom the consultant is responsible, managerial duties, agreed commitments outside the trust etc.). The reasons for consultants having less than seven fixed commitments should

Exhibit 23
Improving the use of job plans

Job plans should be comprehensive, consistent, monitored and regularly reviewed.

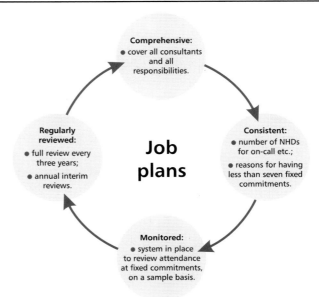

Source: Audit Commission.

be clear. The mix of commitments should vary according to the needs of the service and training and to accommodate the changing interests and skills of consultants over their working lives.

Monitored

78. Trusts should ensure that consultants comply with their job plans. For activities such as teaching, audit and management, the emphasis should be on achievements and standards. However, for fixed commitments trusts should monitor consultants' attendance. This can be done on a sample basis and should be carried out sensitively. The majority of consultants fulfil their fixed commitments and need have nothing to fear from such monitoring. In the very few cases where disciplinary proceedings become necessary, detailed information will be needed about an individual's commitments (from the job plans) and their performance. Many disciplinary actions fail at the moment for lack of this detail (Ref. 27). Trusts should be able to monitor compliance with job plans using data on the use of operating theatres and outpatient clinics, such as that in Exhibits 21 and 22. Many trusts already collect this data, but do not process it. The Audit Commission's auditors will be assisting trusts to do this over the next year.

79. Trusts also have a duty to ask whole-time consultants to state their income from private practice each year (to monitor the 'ten-per-cent-of-income' rule, see page 44) and to assure themselves that maximum-part-time consultants are *'...devoting substantially the whole of their professional time to the NHS'* (Ref. 23). Private practice done outside normal NHS hours may compromise the quality of NHS patient care if it results in a consultant being too tired as a result of overworking.

Regularly reviewed

80. The national guidelines suggest that job plans should be reviewed annually. This should take place in a face-to-face meeting between the consultant and the appropriate manager (ideally the clinical director). It should provide an opportunity to discuss the consultant's job satisfaction and training needs, as well as to consider changes in emphasis in a consultant's work programme as his or her career progresses. In most hospitals there are too many consultants for a chief executive to see each one personally. Medical and clinical directors need to become involved in job plan reviews and in their original specification. The involvement of clinical directors should also facilitate a closer correspondence between job plans and a trust's service and training commitments. Appropriate management arrangements for doctors is the key to achieving change in this as in many other areas of medical staffing. It is discussed further in Chapter 5.

More even distribution of the work

81. Within specialties the work should be distributed as evenly as possible between the consultants involved. This can be achieved partly by changes in the referral system (previously discussed – page 28) and partly through a review of each individual's workload, particularly the balance between clinical and non-clinical work. Even though many consultants work beyond their contracted hours, it is essential to ensure that they are contributing fully in terms of fixed commitments and meeting their training obligations and are not being overburdened by pressure of work in other areas. In some hospitals the attendance of full-time consultants at only two or less outpatient clinics or two or less theatre sessions per week suggests that there is scope for increasing their clinical work.

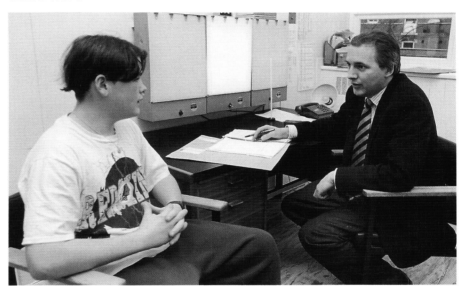

Recommendations for NHS trusts on the contribution of consultants

1   Job plans must be completed for all consultants and specify all their duties and responsibilities.

2   The number of each consultant's fixed commitments should be set according to agreed rules. These rules should be consistent for all consultants working in a specialty or trust and give explicit reasons for less than seven fixed commitments.

3   Trusts should monitor consultants' compliance with these commitments, probably on a sample basis.

4   Trusts should assure themselves that there are no conflicts between NHS and private work.

5   Job plans should be reviewed at least annually. Clinical directors should play a greater role in the review process than they do at the moment and link it to service and training commitments.

6   The workload of a specialty should be more evenly distributed between consultants. The balance between clinical and non-clinical work of individual consultants should be reviewed. In some cases more clinical work may be justified.

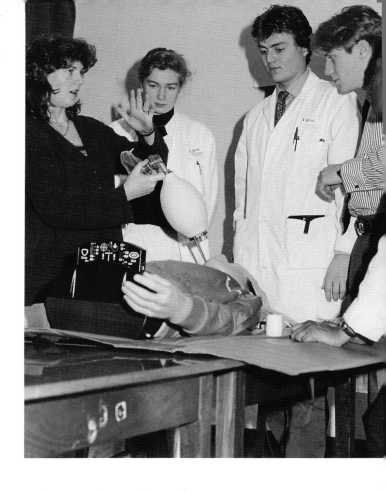

4 The Organisation and Management of Training

The national guidelines on postgraduate medical training make provision for each trainee to have an educational supervisor, a personal training programme and to be properly assessed, but these provisions are often not met locally. Training structures are based largely on 'inputs', such as time spent, rather than achievements and there is relatively little scope for part-time training for which a candidate still has to demonstrate special needs. Few trusts have a policy for the continuing professional development of their career grade doctors and the average amount of study leave taken is well below the level allowed in national terms and conditions of service.

Trusts need to establish more effective arrangements for managing training which include clearer responsibilities and more consistency of approach, where appropriate, between the specialties. More structured training programmes should be introduced, including longer contracts consisting of a series of linked posts. More part-time posts are needed with less bureaucracy for doctors to obtain them. More opportunities for professional development should be provided.

'Training is now very much at a turning point'

82. The role of NHS hospitals in training clinical staff is second only in importance to their role in providing patient care. Most, if not all, acute hospitals in England and Wales undertake postgraduate training of doctors. Even doctors who are planning a career in general practice must spend at least two years training in hospital. The need to take training requirements into account when making decisions about the skill mix and deployment of doctors has been stressed in Chapter 2. This chapter is concerned with the organisation and management of the training itself.

83. Training is now very much at a turning point. The structuring of medical staffing into firms and the associated unwritten rules have had as big an influence on training as they have on the skill mix and deployment of doctors. Medical royal colleges and their training committees are still responsible for inspecting and approving all NHS training posts, but postgraduate deans now have a major role in the organisation of training locally. They hold budgets to cover 50 per cent of the basic salary costs of all training grade posts and agree contracts for training with each trust, thus influencing the number of training posts trusts have. In doing so they must consider the aims of the local health care purchasers and coordinate their role with that of the royal colleges. All parties have to ensure that the right balance is struck between service quality and efficiency, on the one hand, and the need to train and develop doctors for the future on the other.

84. Changes in the conduct of training are already underway in response to *Achieving a Balance* and the *New Deal* which have sought to increase the amount of patient care provided by career grades and reduce junior doctors' hours of work. Implementation of the Calman report is resulting in more explicit training curricula. Attachment of trainees to individual consultants is being replaced by attachment to teams so that in the course of a single post junior doctors can expect to receive training from several consultants. And a debate is beginning about the correct balance of locating medical training between hospitals and the community they serve. In these circumstances the need for clear and consistent training standards and policies at hospital level is particularly important.

The problems

Inadequate management of postgraduate training

85. The GMC and the medical royal colleges have laid down firm guidelines on the content and management of postgraduate medical training. The four key principles included in the guidelines are:

- **Proper induction training at the take up of a post.** The majority of doctors attend induction courses covering the hospital in general (and a large minority do not), but they are much less likely to attend sessions on the way their specialty is practised in that hospital. And senior training grade doctors are much less likely to attend these events than are the junior grades (Exhibit 24). Although most hospitals say they arrange such sessions, they seldom collect data on uptake. It is therefore unclear whether the problems relate to lack of provision or lack of uptake.

- **Appointment of an educational supervisor.** Forty-six per cent of junior doctors at the hospitals studied by the Audit Commission said they did not have an educational supervisor, and there was much confusion about the meaning of this term. The GMC and royal colleges' guidelines require that all trainees should have a consultant as an educational supervisor but, of those who said they did have a supervisor, some referred to another training grade doctor (e.g. registrar).

- **Agreement of a training programme to meet the specific needs of the trainee.** Most consultants at the study sites stated that they discuss personal training needs with their juniors, but only a third of juniors at the same hospitals concurred with this view (Exhibit 25, overleaf). Most of those who did discuss training ended up agreeing a training programme.

Exhibit 24
Doctors' attendance at induction courses

Most junior doctors attend induction courses for the hospital, but few attend a course or a session for their specialty.

Sample size: 207.

Source: Audit Commission.

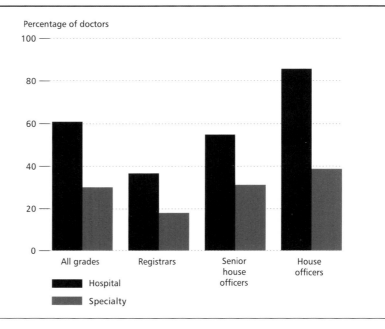

Percentage of doctors

■ Hospital
■ Specialty

Exhibit 25
Training programmes for junior doctors

Most junior doctors do not have personal training programmes.

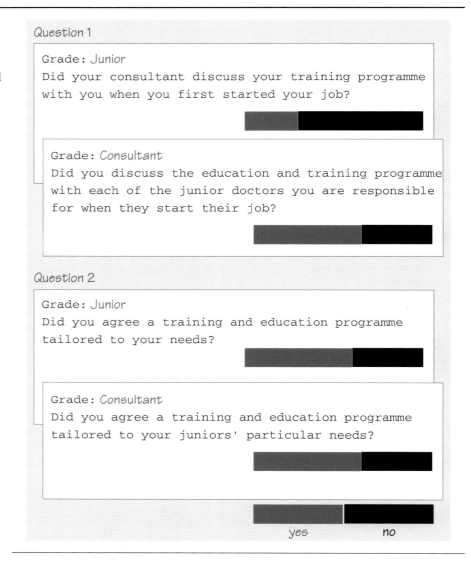

Question 1

Grade: Junior
Did your consultant discuss your training programme with you when you first started your job?

Grade: Consultant
Did you discuss the education and training programme with each of the junior doctors you are responsible for when they start their job?

Question 2

Grade: Junior
Did you agree a training and education programme tailored to your needs?

Grade: Consultant
Did you agree a training and education programme tailored to your juniors' particular needs?

yes   no

Sample size: 201.

Source: Audit Commission.

◆ **Proper assessment and appraisal.** Eighty-five per cent of consultants at the study sites said they had at least one meeting with juniors whilst they were in post, but only 45 per cent of junior doctors said this was the case. Only a quarter of the consultants claimed to give written feedback to juniors on their performance. Junior doctors, particularly those in the most junior grades, reported that their clinical skills were not routinely assessed even though they employ many of these skills independently (Exhibit 26).

Exhibit 26
Assessment of clinical skills

All doctors in training, and particularly the most junior, report that their clinical skills are not routinely assessed.

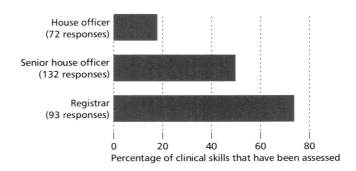

Percentage of clinical skills that have been assessed

Note: each doctor was asked which of three basic clinical skills (according to grade and specialty listed below) they undertook unsupervised. Those who answered 'yes' were then asked whether their competence to carry out the skills had ever been assessed? The proportion of skills undertaken that had not been assessed was then calculated for the whole sample.

Specialty / grade	House officer	Senior house officer	Registrar
General medicine	Set up intravenous line	Central venous line insertion	Insert a temporary cardiac pacing wire
	Manage an acute asthma attack	Chest drain insertion	Chest drain insertion
	Manage a patient in clinical shock	Lumbar puncture	Gastro-intestinal endoscopy or bronchoscopy
General surgery	Manage the acute abdomen	Elective hernia repair	Perform an elective bowel resection
	Manage a post-operative patient in clinical shock	Emergency appendectomy	Operate on a strangulated hernia
	Carry out minor operations, e.g. 'lumps and bumps'	Manage the acutely painful testicle	Manage acute trauma
Obstetrics and gynaecology		Manage a case of vaginal bleeding in early pregnancy	Manage a case of acute pregnancy-induced hypertension (pre-eclampsia)
		Perform a diagnostic dilatation and curettage	Perform a lower segment caesarean section
		Suture an episiotomy	Perform a breech delivery
Ear, nose and throat		Perform indirect laryngoscopy	Perform direct (rigid) laryngoscopy
		Perform a tonsillectomy on a child	Carry out mastoid cavity surgery
		Manage epistaxis	Perform a tracheotomy

Source: Audit Commission.

86. Most clinical skills need to be formally taught and assessed; and some should be regularly reviewed to make sure that they are maintained. Cardio-pulmonary resuscitation (CPR) skills, for example, once taught, should ideally be reviewed about every six months (Ref. 28). Most hospitals provide some CPR training, but few systematically ensure that reviews take place. Ninety-five per cent of junior doctors surveyed had received some training in CPR, but on average it had been 22 months earlier. Only 40 per cent of the sample had received training in their current hospital, and of those only a half had had their skills formally assessed (Exhibit 27).

Inflexible training structures

87. Doctors undertaking postgraduate training face other problems with training structures:

◆ **Assessment is based heavily on inputs.** Most specialties have formal college examinations in the middle of the training period, after which trainees progress by following specific paths and spend particular amounts of time at the various stages.

◆ **Lack of scope for part-time training.** Far too few posts are currently available on a part-time basis and doctors have to justify special needs to obtain them (Exhibit 28). Though the controls in the system have just been devolved from national committees to regional level (Ref. 29), it can still involve considerable bureaucracy and make it very difficult to move between full-time and part-time posts. Demand for part-time training posts has declined, perhaps because many doctors are apparently not aware of the arrangements for obtaining them (Ref. 16). Many doctors also feel that part-time training does not carry the same weight as full-time training.

Exhibit 27
Training in cardio-pulmonary resuscitation

Most hospitals provide some CPR training, but many do not systematically ensure that reviews take place.

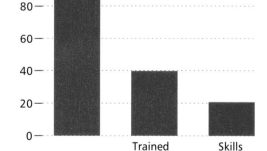

Percentage of junior doctors

Sample size: 174.

Source: Audit Commission.

Exhibit 28
Part-time posts in the training grades

Far too few posts are currently available
on a part-time basis.

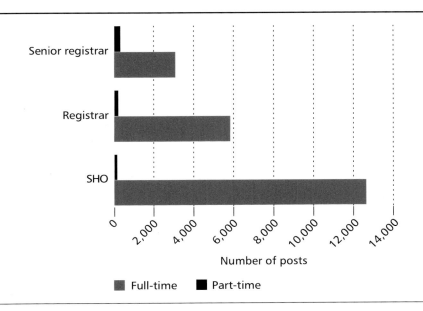

Number of posts

Full-time   Part-time

*Source: Department of Health Medical Manpower
Statistics.*

88. The need to move around the country continually in pursuit of hospital medical training was identified by many doctors, regardless of gender, as leading to problems in their personal relationships and social lives (Ref. 16).

Lack of professional development for career grade staff

89. It is now accepted that continuing education and training are necessary for doctors in all the career grades. Such training needs to cover managerial and organisational matters as well as clinical developments. So it is unfortunate that in some hospitals there is little opportunity for training, and in others the opportunity exists but the uptake is low. Whether the cause is lack of interest or lack of funding, the outcome is the same. At the study sites consultants took an average of only six days study leave per year (30 days in any period of three years is the maximum allowed in the national terms and conditions of service – Ref. 23). The picture for staff grade doctors is much the same (Ref. 17). But the quantity of study leave is only part of the picture. It is important that the study leave is used appropriately and productively and few trusts monitor that.

Overcoming the problems

Improving the management of post graduate training

90. The purchaser/provider split in postgraduate medical training sets clear local responsibilities for specifying and implementing training. Postgraduate deans should seize the opportunity jointly with NHS trusts and purchasers to bring improvements to many long-standing training problems. All NHS trust boards must accept that they have a major responsibility for medical training. And all trusts need to develop a medical training strategy, based on the training contract (Exhibit 29). The strategy should include:

◆ **Clear responsibilities for training**. The medical director is accountable to the trust board on training issues and the clinical tutor, as local agent of the post graduate dean, is responsible for co-ordinating training. Each clinical directorate or specialty needs to have one consultant with overall responsibility for training policy and every trainee should have a personal training supervisor.

◆ **Coordination across the hospital of training activities and standards.** One approach is to set up a training committee, probably chaired by the clinical tutor but with the medical director and specialty tutors, appointed by the relevant royal college, as members. This committee could then:

– develop policies and procedures for formal training to include induction courses (induction courses for HOs became compulsory in August 1994 – Ref. 30), training and assessment of CPR skills and the production of a doctors' handbook (Exhibit 30);

Exhibit 29
Implementation of a training strategy

Trusts need to develop a medical training strategy, based on the training contract.

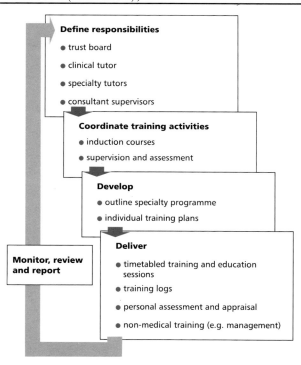

Define responsibilities
● trust board
● clinical tutor
● specialty tutors
● consultant supervisors

Coordinate training activities
● induction courses
● supervision and assessment

Develop
● outline specialty programme
● individual training plans

Deliver
● timetabled training and education sessions
● training logs
● personal assessment and appraisal
● non-medical training (e.g. management)

Monitor, review and report

Source: Audit Commission.

– agree consistent approaches to issues such as the nature of training programmes for individual doctors, and methods of supervision and assessment – e.g. training logs to record work done and assessment of

Exhibit 30
Model contents of a junior doctor's handbook

All junior doctors should be given a handbook when they take up a new post.

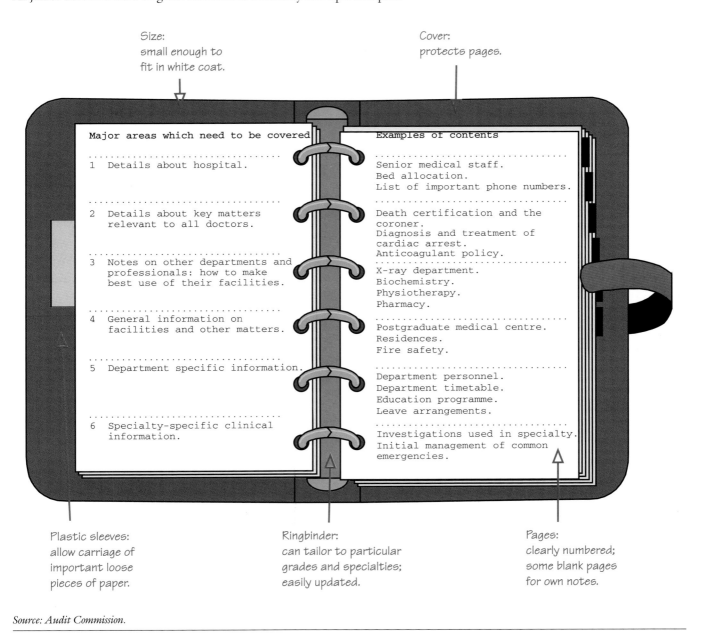

Size:
small enough to
fit in white coat.

Cover:
protects pages.

Major areas which need to be covered | Examples of contents

1 Details about hospital.
Senior medical staff.
Bed allocation.
List of important phone numbers.

2 Details about key matters relevant to all doctors.
Death certification and the coroner.
Diagnosis and treatment of cardiac arrest.
Anticoagulant policy.

3 Notes on other departments and professionals: how to make best use of their facilities.
X-ray department.
Biochemistry.
Physiotherapy.
Pharmacy.

4 General information on facilities and other matters.
Postgraduate medical centre.
Residences.
Fire safety.

5 Department specific information.
Department personnel.
Department timetable.
Education programme.
Leave arrangements.

6 Specialty-specific clinical information.
Investigations used in specialty.
Initial management of common emergencies.

Plastic sleeves:
allow carriage of
important loose
pieces of paper.

Ringbinder:
can tailor to particular
grades and specialties;
easily updated.

Pages:
clearly numbered;
some blank pages
for own notes.

Source: Audit Commission.

skills such as those developed by the Royal College of Ophthalmologists for SHOs can assist in this process (Ref. 31);

– monitor and review progress regularly and report annually to the trust board.

91. Postgraduate deans are already developing detailed rules and guidance for doctors as part of their training contracts (Exhibit 31) which could also be incorporated into doctors' handbooks. This is a welcome development. A training coordinating committee would put trusts in a stronger position to implement these.

Providing more flexible training

92. Individual trainees need a more structured approach to their training. Doctors and managers in NHS trusts need clearer guidance on how they should assess the competence of individual doctors. Improvements in the specification and monitoring of training programmes for higher specialist

---

Exhibit 31
Junior doctors' information leaflet

Some postgraduate deans are already developing detailed rules and guidance for trainees.

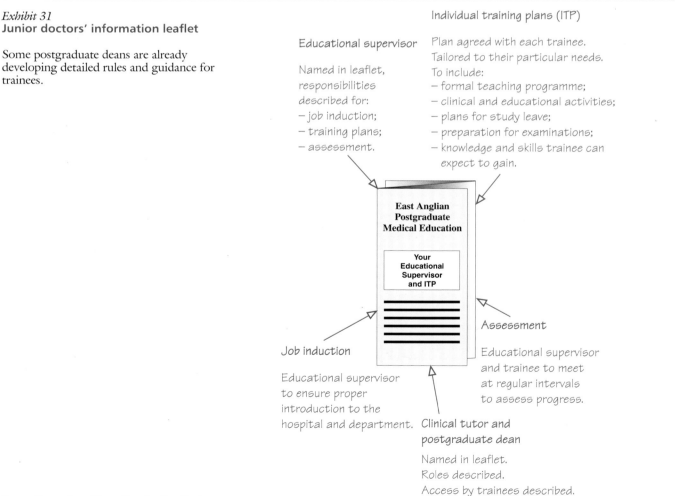

Individual training plans (ITP)

Educational supervisor

Named in leaflet, responsibilities described for:
– job induction;
– training plans;
– assessment.

Plan agreed with each trainee.
Tailored to their particular needs.
To include:
– formal teaching programme;
– clinical and educational activities;
– plans for study leave;
– preparation for examinations;
– knowledge and skills trainee can expect to gain.

East Anglian Postgraduate Medical Education

Your Educational Supervisor and ITP

Job induction

Educational supervisor to ensure proper introduction to the hospital and department.

Assessment

Educational supervisor and trainee to meet at regular intervals to assess progress.

Clinical tutor and postgraduate dean

Named in leaflet.
Roles described.
Access by trainees described.

Source: Postgraduate Dean, East Anglian Region.

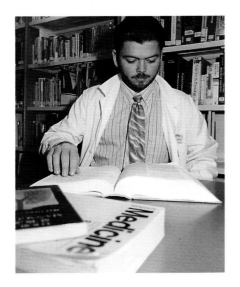

trainees are already underway as part of the implementation of the Calman report. This is a welcome development because it directs the emphasis in medical training firmly in favour of 'outputs', i.e. what the training should achieve, and away from 'inputs' such as a trainee's timetable, which are only a means to the end. Similar guidelines are needed for SHOs and HOs.

93. For many doctors training consists of an uncoordinated series of posts, at least until they reach registrar level, even though four fifths of doctors who left medical school in 1986 say they would prefer training programmes with predetermined rotations of posts (Ref. 16). Some trusts already have SHO posts that last two years or more where trainees agree to work in the same hospital (or in a number of hospitals with a joint arrangement) pursuing a clear course of training developed as part of a single contract. Others should seek to introduce such arrangements with the cooperation of postgraduate deans. Longer-term posts also lead to fewer appointment committees and consequently lower costs for the NHS.

94. More opportunities should be provided for part-time training. The bureaucracy involved in obtaining approval to work in a part-time post and in taking a career break needs to be drastically reduced. A five per cent increase in the number of part-time training posts by the end of the century has recently been recommended (Ref. 32), but it is doubtful whether this will be enough. More job-sharing schemes could be introduced. Doctors working part-time sometimes claim that the quality and extent of training they receive may be greater than that of their full-time counterparts for the same number of hours on duty and if assessment were based more on achievement they would be able to demonstrate this and thereby increase the status of part-time training. The Government and the royal colleges should urgently review training standards and guidelines with a view to increasing the number of part-time posts and providing greater flexibility for trainees in other ways.

Continuing professional development

95. Policies for the professional development of consultants and staff grade doctors should be part of trusts' training plans. Trusts are responsible for funding study leave and should ensure that it is relevant to the needs of the service as well as the professional needs of the individuals concerned. They should also have a separately earmarked budget.

96. Several of the royal colleges are proposing systems of specialist re-certification based on the need to acquire points for educational activities approved by the colleges. The formal recognition of the need for and content of continuing medical education is a welcome step forward, but it does need to be set alongside priorities for consultants' and staff grade doctors' non-medical training needs such as management and communication skills.

Recommendations on the organisation and management of training

Trusts

1 Every trust should have a training strategy in place which:

- sets out the responsibilities of all staff concerned with training; and
- gives the trust's broad approach to training issues such as induction of new doctors, responsibilities of training supervisors and methods of assessment and appraisal.

2 Each individual trainee doctor should have a consultant supervisor whose main tasks are:

- to agree a training programme specific to the needs of that doctor;
- monitor the doctor's progress; and
- provide feedback and assessment.

3 Every trust should have a policy for the continuing professional development of career grade doctors as part of its training strategy. This should include non-medical as well as medical training needs and reflect the priorities of the trust as well as those of the individual doctors concerned.

Other bodies

4 The **royal colleges** should set definite standards which trainees at all levels must meet. These standards are vital not only to training but to patient care as well.

5 **Postgraduate deans in cooperation with the royal colleges and NHS trusts** should develop more structured training programmes for doctors including contracts covering a series of linked posts.

6 The **Government, the royal colleges and individual trusts** should reduce the bureaucracy involved for trainees seeking part-time work and increase the number of part-time posts. More job-sharing schemes are needed.

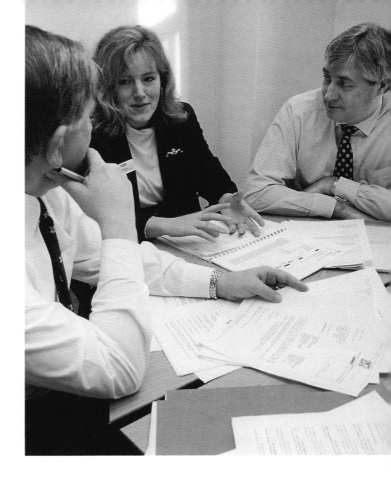

5 A Framework for Change

As the recommendations in the report are implemented, the need for such close control of individual posts and the number of doctors at each grade by the national bodies should diminish. But placing greater control in the hands of individual trusts does require a much closer working relationship between doctors and managers and for doctors to become more involved in the management of their own work. Clinical directors have a key role to play in this.

97. The quality of medical care individual patients receive in NHS hospitals depends, to a large extent, on the doctors responsible for their diagnosis and treatment. The mix of skills and working practices, standards of supervision, training and continuing professional education are all important factors.

98. This report has demonstrated the considerable complexity in organising hospital doctors' work. Three factors underpin this complexity:

◆ several national bodies have influence over the numbers of grades and posts in particular hospitals and over the standards and requirements for training;

◆ there is a need to reconcile two different and sometimes conflicting sets of responsibilities: the responsibility to deliver a high quality of care to patients as efficiently as possible, whilst at the same time planning and delivering high quality medical training to junior doctors; and

◆ it is difficult to change doctors' working practices because they have evolved over a long period of time, are informal and need to be formal and are deeply rooted in the culture, custom and practice of hospitals.

99. Each of the preceding chapters has examined the problems and, where possible, made recommendations on specific aspects of medical staffing. Implementing any of these recommendations will, however, require the right conditions:

◆ appropriate national controls;

◆ incentives to give doctors at all levels in trusts a reason for their involvement; and

◆ clearer and more positive relationships between managers and doctors.

Appropriate national controls on medical staffing

100. There is considerable external control of trusts on medical staffing matters. At the moment the Department of Health and the Welsh Office regulate the number of doctors in most grades – other than consultant – at national level and, in some cases, at regional level as well. The royal colleges (the bodies responsible for both general professional and higher specialist training) have a variety of influences. They inspect and approve individual posts and they have representation on consultant appointment committees. As many of the changes outlined in this report begin to take effect, such control should be re-evaluated. With clear guidelines on skills and tasks appropriate to each grade so that trusts are unable to employ either trainee doctors or staff grade doctors to substitute inappropriately for the work of consultants, it may prove possible to remove some of the controls on the number of posts. In this context the Audit Commission welcomes the Government's decision to produce guidance on 'medical staff-mix and skill-mix' (Ref. 33).

Incentives for doctors at all levels

101. Many of the recommendations in this report will offer advantages to doctors as well as resulting in more efficient and effective organisation of medical staffing. Improvements in the organisation and management of medical training, for example, will bring direct benefits to individuals. But what incentives are there to change long-standing working arrangements? The

' Many of the recommendations in this report will offer advantages to doctors as well as resulting in more efficient and effective organisation of medical staffing'

most important is a pressure for change from recently qualified doctors. They are no longer prepared to be part of some 'lost tribe', nor to work long unsocial hours and frequently move around the country in pursuit of a medical career at the expense of their personal lives. Doctors who have gone through this process sometimes look back on it as part of an initiation, but now there are external pressures for change as well. The national initiatives on medical staffing and the increasing role of trust managers in medical staffing are important examples. In addition, the Audit Commission's auditors will be assisting acute hospital trusts over the next year to assess their individual needs for change in medical staffing and to develop action plans.

102. NHS trusts have freedom to employ new consultants largely on whatever terms and conditions they wish. To date very few trusts have departed from the national terms and conditions of service, particularly as a result of opposition from doctors, but also because the continued existence of a strong national pay review body and recent limitations on public sector pay have all restricted their scope for action (Ref. 34). Local pay incentives might attract some doctors to particular posts but should be set against the risk that the overall pay bill of NHS doctors might rise and that it might become more difficult to attract doctors to areas of work or locations which could not meet the premiums offered elsewhere.

103. Distinction awards are a national system of performance pay for consultants. The scheme, which is under review, was set up at the inception of the NHS. It is currently outside the control of individual trusts although they must meet its financial consequences. Consultants are nominated for distinction awards by regional committees consisting mainly of doctors. Decisions on whether to make the awards are taken nationally for the top awards (A+, A and B) and regionally for the lower ones (C awards). They vary in value from 20 per cent of basic salary for a C award (about £10,000) to 100 per cent for an A+ award (about £47,000 – Ref. 35) and they are superannuable. The criteria for awards vary according to the category and include: 'clinical excellence and recognition of leadership'; 'outstanding administrative or management effort'; or simply 'hard work and outstanding service to the NHS which may alone be sufficient for recognition' (Ref. 35). Since 1989 awards have been subject to review every five years and, at least in theory, this can result in their downgrading or removal. The Government has recently published a report which recommends clearer separation into local and national awards, greater involvement of NHS employers in local awards and 'top-sliced' or central funding for higher awards (Ref. 36). The Audit Commission welcomes these recommendations but, given the large sums of public money involved (£104m in 1993/94 – Ref. 35), considers there is a need for trust managers to have an unconditional veto on local awards, since they affect the trust budget, and for these awards to be of limited duration, renewal being subject to the doctor continuing to meet the criteria.

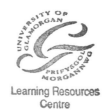

Clearer and more positive relationships between doctors and managers

104. There is a need for more active involvement of doctors in the management of their work and in that of the trust as a whole. NHS trusts have a non-executive chairman and up to five non-executive directors and five executive directors. One of the five executive directors will be the medical director. Clinical directors are often organised into a lower level board along with other senior executives, and consultants often have a separate medical advisory committee. The routes through which doctors can influence trust policy and trust boards can communicate their plans to the doctors who deliver them are frequently not clear. Many of the issues and problems raised in this report will only be solved if trust boards take responsibility on themselves for ensuring the right cultural climate and framework for action (Box 3).

105. Clinical directors should play a major role in the trust management process and particularly in medical staffing issues. It will often be more appropriate for the clinical director to provide the lead on staffing issues rather than for individual consultants because they are best placed to assess patient care and training needs in the directorate as a whole. Clinical directorates were to have been the main mechanism for managing staff and activity, but in practice they are often only mechanisms for managing budgets. Clinical directors do not have managerial authority over the consultants in their directorates nor over the junior doctors: the perception of consultants as autonomous and juniors as 'belonging' to them continues in many hospitals. Trusts need to develop more effective ways of holding individual consultants to account (e.g. for fixed commitments) and more consistent policies for managing junior doctors through clinical directorates. Clinical directors should be key players for implementing many of the recommendations in this report (Box 4).

Box 3
The role of the trust board

The whole board should:

◆ ensure that the trust agrees on the mechanisms for managing doctors and their role in patient care and medical training.

The chief executive should:

◆ implement the agreements reached by the trust board and ensure that regular monitoring and review take place.

The medical director should:

◆ be medical adviser to the trust board;

◆ communicate trust policy to the clinical directors and consultants;

◆ take strategic responsibility for issues such as conditions of service for medical staff, consultant appointment procedures, medical audit and postgraduate medical training strategy (the latter in coordination with the clinical tutor); and

◆ coordinate and prioritise proposals from doctors to the trust board.

Box 4
Elements of the clinical director's role

- Implementation of service and training contracts.
- Medical staff planning (e.g. skill mix of doctors and deployment).
- Consultant job plans – specification and review.
- Accountability of consultants for fixed commitments.
- Continuing medical education and other training for consultants and staff grade doctors.
- Directorate policies on junior doctors' hours of work, supervision, tasks and responsibilities.
- Implementation of medical and clinical audit.
- Development of management guidelines and protocols for clinical procedures.
- Specialty level induction and information packs for new doctors.

106. Trusts must make time available for clinical directors' management duties. There may be compensating reductions in other managers' time. Seventy-two per cent of clinical directors have between one and two sessions per week set aside for their management duties, but in practice 70 per cent spend more time than this (Ref. 37).

107. Although this report has looked separately at skill mix and deployment, the contribution of consultants and the organisation and management of training, the three areas are clearly interlinked. Doctors and trust managers need to recognise this and work together to implement the recommendations in a comprehensive and coordinated way. For too long specific medical staffing issues have been thought to be the province just of doctors or of managers, or even of bodies outside hospitals altogether, and dealt with far too narrowly. There is now an opportunity, indeed a necessity, for all trusts to review their management arrangements and the roles of their medical staff.

Action checklist

1 Trusts should:

- clarify the roles of doctors and other professions;
- specify the required nature and extent of supervision of junior doctors;
- encourage consultants to share the workload more evenly;
- deploy doctors more efficiently in relation to service and training needs;
- introduce policies and more posts to take account of the special needs of doctors with family commitments;
- ensure that job plans are complete for all consultants and are regularly reviewed;
- aim for each consultant to undertake seven fixed commitments – the reasons for a lower number being accepted should be made explicit;
- ensure that all doctors in training have proper training programmes and that the programmes are regularly monitored and assessed;
- develop a policy for the continuing professional development of career grade doctors;
- implement these recommendations through a medical staffing plan and training strategy with clearly defined responsibilities for action; and
- encourage doctors to take a more active role in management, particularly clinical directors, and in medical staffing issues.

2 Regional postgraduate deans should:

- develop detailed polices on the nature and extent of supervision of junior doctors;
- develop more structured training programmes for doctors in collaboration with the royal colleges;
- aim to introduce policies and more posts to take account of the special needs of doctors with family commitments;
- ensure that junior doctors have access to good careers advice; and
- ensure that junior doctors' working conditions, especially the on-call facilities, are of a sufficiently high standard.

3   The Department of Health and the Welsh Office should:

- produce guidance on the appropriate grade and skill mix of doctors as soon as possible;
- review the need for national controls on the number of posts at different grades as training and competence requirements become more explicit;
- reduce the bureaucracy involved in training part-time and increase the number of part-time posts; and
- monitor the changing roles of the medical profession and ensure that training structures and processes adapt to reflect them.

4   The royal colleges should:

- set definite standards for the competence of junior doctors at all levels;
- encourage the development of more structured training programmes;
- reduce the bureaucracy involved in training part-time;
- change the way they monitor training so that it focuses much more on 'outputs' or achievements, rather than 'inputs';
- publicise the advice schemes they already have in place for career advice and introduce new ones; and
- monitor the changing roles of the medical profession and ensure that training structures and processes adapt to reflect them.

Appendix 1 – Acknowledgements

The study sites

The following NHS trusts assisted with data collection in the study:

Bassetlaw Hospital and Community Services

City Hospitals, Sunderland

East Hertfordshire Health, Welwyn Garden City

Freeman Group of Hospitals, Newcastle-upon-Tyne

Gateshead Hospitals

Glan Clwyd District General Hospital, Rhyl

Good Hope Hospital, Sutton Coldfield, Birmingham

Gwynedd Hospitals, Bangor

Harrogate Health Care

Leicester General Hospital

Mid-Essex Hospital Services

North Middlesex Hospital

North Tees Health, Stockton-on-Tees

Northwick Park and St Mark's, Harrow

Poole Hospital

Riverside Hospitals, London

Royal Liverpool University Hospital

South Buckinghamshire, High Wycombe

South Devon Healthcare, Torquay

Southport and Formby

St George's, London

St James's University Hospital, Leeds

Taunton and Somerset

The Addenbrooke's, Cambridge

The Royal Free Hampstead

Worthing and Southlands Hospitals

The advisory group

The following were members of the advisory group:

Mr S. Brearley, Consultant Surgeon, Whipps Cross Hospital, London

Mr C. Bulstrode, Clinical Reader in Orthopaedic Surgery, John Radcliffe Hospital, Oxford

Mr S. Catling, Assistant Secretary, Department of Health

Mr A. Christopher, Audit Commission

Dr Robin Dowie, Senior Research Fellow, British Postgraduate Medical Federation

Sir Terence English, Consultant Surgeon, Papworth Hospital, Cambridge and Audit Commission

Dr Ruth Gilbert, Lecturer in Epidemiology, Institute of Child Health, London

Professor A Maynard, Director of the Centre for Health Economics, University of York

Mr N. McKay, Chief Executive, Northern General Hospital NHS Trust, Sheffield

Dr M. McKee, Senior Lecturer in Public Health, London School of Hygiene and Tropical Medicine

Dr Elizabeth Shore, Postgraduate Dean (retired), North West Thames RHA

Dr R. Stott, Medical Director, Lewisham NHS Trust

Margaret Wheatcroft, Director of Nursing and Patient Services, Royal Bournemouth Hospital NHS Trust

Mr C. Wilkinson, Audit Commission

Others

Mike Burbidge, Atwork Health Systems, staff of the Freeman Hospital, Newcastle-upon-Tyne and St James's University Hospital, Leeds, assisted with data collection and analysis.

Appendix 2 – The Study Sites

The study sites (listed in Appendix 1) fall into three categories:

- main study sites, where the interviews and questionnaire surveys of doctors were carried out (11 sites – see Appendix 3);

- operating theatre sites which provided data for the analysis of surgeons' NHS workloads (Appendix 4) and private practice (Appendix 5) – ten sites; and

- pilot audit sites where questionnaire surveys were also carried out (Appendix 3) and which provided data on consultants' use of outpatient clinics (Appendix 6) – five sites.

The study sites were selected to include a variety of hospital types and geographical locations (Tables A2.1 and A2.2).

Table A2.1
Hospital type at study sites

	Hospital type		
	Number of teaching hospitals	**Number of non-teaching hospitals**	**Total**
Main study sites	2	9	11
Operating theatre sites	4	6	10
Pilot audit sites	2	3	5

Source: Audit Commission.

Table A2.2
Geographical distribution of study sites

	NHS region					
	North West, Northern and Yorkshire	**Trent, West Midlands**	**Anglia and Oxford, South and West**	**North and South Thames**	**Wales**	**Total**
Main study sites	3	2	2	3	1	11
Operating theatre sites	3	1	2	3	1	10
Pilot audit sites	2	1		2		5

Source: Audit Commission.

Appendix 3 – Questionnaires Sent to Doctors at the Study Sites

The questionnaires were intended mainly to collect information on the organisation of doctors' work, supervision of juniors, allocation of tasks and assessment of clinical skills and training. Revised versions are in use in the local audits now underway.

Nearly 1,100 questionnaires were sent to individual doctors at the main study sites and the pilot audit sites – consultants and juniors. The majority of doctors included are in general medicine, general surgery and obstetrics and gynaecology. The overall response rate was 60 per cent, but it was much higher for pilot audit sites than main study sites as a result of improvements in survey techniques (Table A3.1). In general, the more senior the doctor, the better the response rate (Exhibit A3.1). There were also some small differences in response rates between specialties (Exhibit A3.2, overleaf).

Table A3.1
Questionnaires sent and response rates at study sites

	Total sent	Respondents	Response rate
Main study sites	799	427	53%
Pilot audit sites	299	228	76%
Total	1098	655	60%

Source: Audit Commission.

Exhibit A3.1
Response rates by grade of doctor (main study sites only)

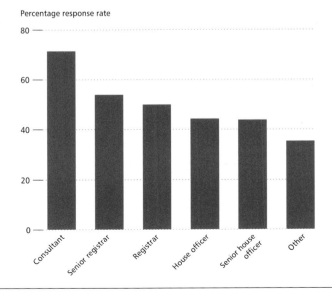

Source: Audit Commission.

Exhibit A3.2
**Response rates by specialty
(main study sites only)**

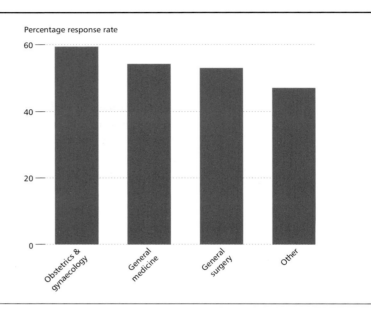

Source: Audit Commission.

The results of the questionnaire surveys are presented in Chapters 2 and 4.

Appendix 4 – NHS Operating Theatre Work

Data routinely available from hospitals usually records operations and procedures for all patients for whom a consultant is responsible, whether or not that consultant was personally involved. They therefore give very little insight into the work of the individual consultant. The main purpose of the data collected from operating theatres in this study was to describe the personal workloads of individual consultants, adjusting for differences in case complexity. It was also used to look at the supervision of junior doctors in operating theatres.

The sample

Ten trusts supplied data (see Appendix 2). Details were obtained of every operation carried out in all specialties by all grades of doctors over a 12-week sample period, 1 April to 30 June 1993. These included: names and grades of surgeon(s) and anaesthetist(s) present, the Office of Population Censuses and Surveys' (OPCS) identifier of the procedure(s) and timings of important events (such as the start and end of the operation). Private operations carried out in NHS operating theatres were excluded where they could be identified. Details of consultants' contracts were obtained separately from medical staffing officers.

Data analysis

The OPCS codes were used to allocate each procedure to one of five categories: minor, intermediate, major, major-plus and complex-major. The categories are defined by private sector insurers for reimbursing doctors and hospitals for their private work and have been used by the Royal College of Surgeons to make recommendations about the workload of consultants (Ref. 38). Average operating times were then derived for each category for each specialty by applying linear regression analysis with the operating time as dependent variable and the number of procedures of each class as independent variables. The operating times are defined as the time 'at the table' (i.e. ignoring the gaps between operations), because this measure was likely to be consistent between sites.

The average operating times calculated, together with the number of procedures on which they are based, are in Table A4.1, overleaf. A separate category ('unknown') was added for the small number of procedures which were not included in the OPCS code-mapping to categories. In addition, hospital-specific averages were used for complex-major operations where their frequencies exceeded 50, because the length of operations was higher for larger hospitals dealing with more complex cases. This resulted in the four teaching hospitals having individual complex-major averages for general surgery, with values ranging from 148 to 196 minutes, compared with the average for other hospitals of 135 minutes.

Table A4.1
Average operating times ('at the table') by category and specialty (minutes)

Specialty	Minor	Intermediate	Major	Major plus	Complex-major	Unknown	Number of procedures in sample
a) Surgical specialties with at least ten consultants in the sample							
General surgery	14	29	53	84	135	40	11,260
Obstetrics and gynaecology	10	11	36	62	88	18	9,610
Otolaryngology	8	20	65	83	109	17	6,589
Trauma and orthopaedics	19	31	52	79	91	32	7,466
Urology	12	24	42	136	193	41	7,054
b) Other surgical specialties							
Dental surgery	25	24	53	93	132	42	2,029
Neuro-surgery	17	44	68	80	95	35	283
Ophthalmology	19	22	26	30	34	39	2,285
Paediatric surgery	21	34	40	70	100	9	241
Plastic surgery	26	34	83	92	131	43	2,475
c) Anaesthetics							
Anaesthetics	14	22	45	73	129	30	49,561

Source: Audit Commission.

These average operating times in the five surgical specialties with at least ten consultants in the sample were used to standardise the weekly output for consultant surgeons in those specialties and arrive at their case-mix-adjusted weekly output. Only consultants on whole-time or maximum-part-time contracts with a single trust are included. No distinction is made between them because the amount of work expected from them is the same. Consultants who were employed by one NHS trust but who also did work for another trust were excluded if that work was not in the sample. The weights for the remaining specialties were used in the comparison of NHS and private work reported in Appendix 5. Comparing the case-mix-adjusted weekly output and the hours actually spent operating ('at the table') gives a measure of a consultant surgeon's speed of operating compared with the average for the specialty as a whole:

- relative speed of operating = case-mix-adjusted weekly output (expressed as 'expected hours') divided by actual time 'at the table' per week (hours).

Various other measures of input were also derived:

- average number of sessions attended per week by consultants (sessions are defined by time of day: 8 a.m. to 1.30 p.m., 1.30 p.m. to 6 p.m.);
- average actual time 'at the table' per session for each consultant.

The number of weeks in the sample was assumed to be ten rather than 12 to allow for an average amount of sickness absence, annual and study leave by the consultants involved.

Results

The results show that the reason some consultants do more work than others is primarily because they operate for more hours, rather than because they work faster. They do more hours mainly because they attend more sessions rather than because their sessions are, on average, longer. The results for the five surgical specialties included are given in exhibits A4.1 to A4.5, overleaf.

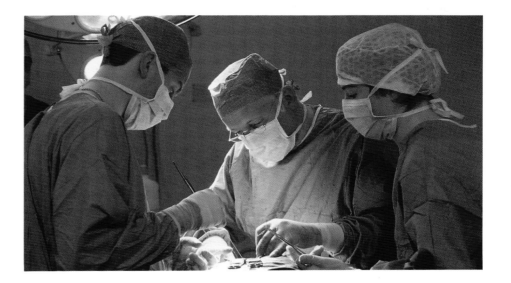

Exhibit A4.1
Consultant surgeons' NHS operating theatre work

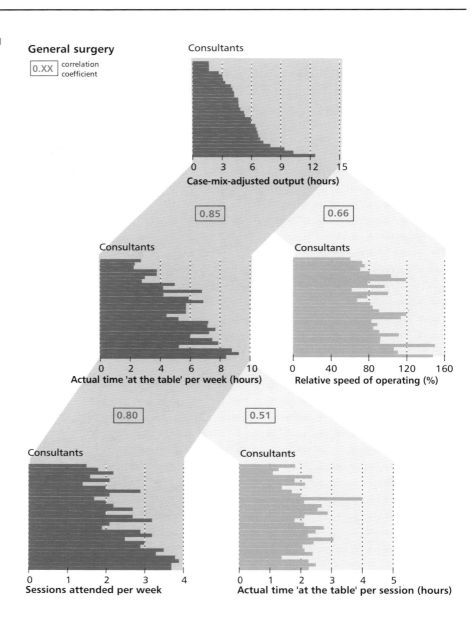

General surgery

0.XX | correlation coefficient

Consultants

0   3   6   9   12   15
Case-mix-adjusted output (hours)

0.85   0.66

Consultants

0   2   4   6   8   10
Actual time 'at the table' per week (hours)

Consultants

0   40   80   120   160
Relative speed of operating (%)

0.80   0.51

Consultants

0   1   2   3   4
Sessions attended per week

Consultants

0   1   2   3   4   5
Actual time 'at the table' per session (hours)

Note: Each bar represents one consultant. They are consistently ordered in each graph, based on case-mix-adjusted weekly output.

Source: Audit Commission.

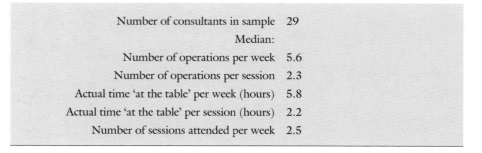

Number of consultants in sample	29
Median:	
Number of operations per week	5.6
Number of operations per session	2.3
Actual time 'at the table' per week (hours)	5.8
Actual time 'at the table' per session (hours)	2.2
Number of sessions attended per week	2.5

Exhibit A4.2
Consultant surgeons' NHS operating theatre work

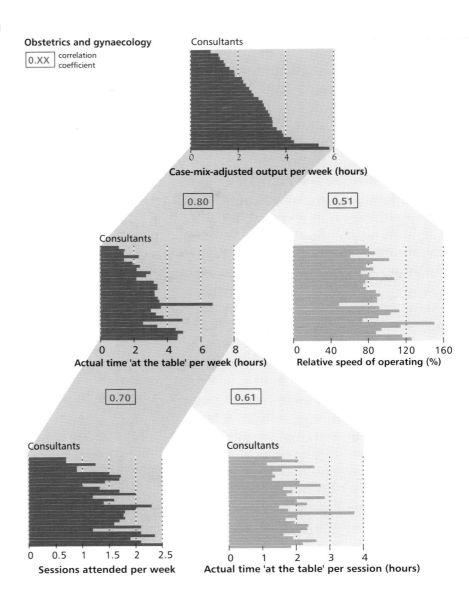

Note: Each bar represents one consultant. They are consistently ordered in each graph, based on case-mix-adjusted weekly output.

Source: Audit Commission.

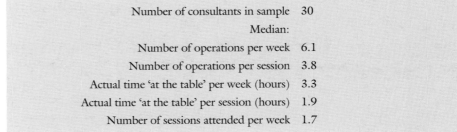

Number of consultants in sample	30
Median:	
Number of operations per week	6.1
Number of operations per session	3.8
Actual time 'at the table' per week (hours)	3.3
Actual time 'at the table' per session (hours)	1.9
Number of sessions attended per week	1.7

Exhibit A4.3
Consultant surgeons' NHS operating
theatre work

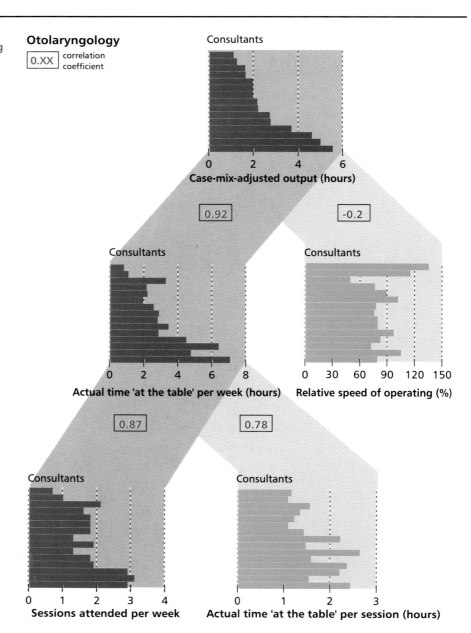

Otolaryngology

0.XX correlation coefficient

Note: Each bar represents one
consultant. They are consistently ordered
in each graph, based on
case-mix-adjusted weekly output.

Source: Audit Commission.

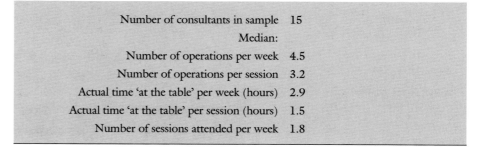

Number of consultants in sample	15
Median:	
Number of operations per week	4.5
Number of operations per session	3.2
Actual time 'at the table' per week (hours)	2.9
Actual time 'at the table' per session (hours)	1.5
Number of sessions attended per week	1.8

Exhibit A4.4
Consultant surgeons' NHS operating theatre work

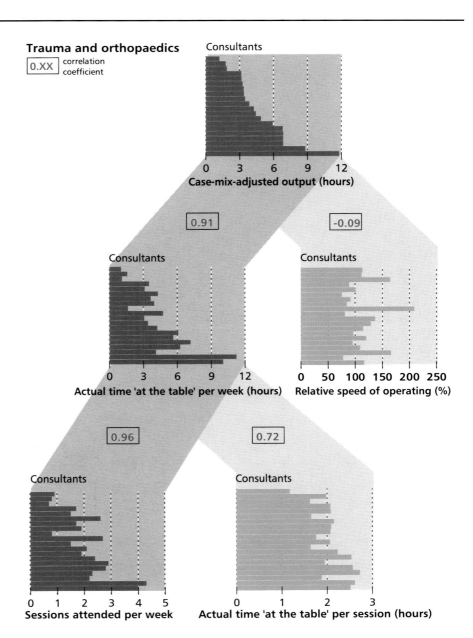

Trauma and orthopaedics

0.XX = correlation coefficient

Consultants

Case-mix-adjusted output (hours)
0 3 6 9 12

0.91   -0.09

Consultants   Consultants

Actual time 'at the table' per week (hours)   **Relative speed of operating (%)**
0 3 6 9 12   0 50 100 150 200 250

0.96   0.72

Consultants   Consultants

Sessions attended per week   **Actual time 'at the table' per session (hours)**
0 1 2 3 4 5   0 1 2 3

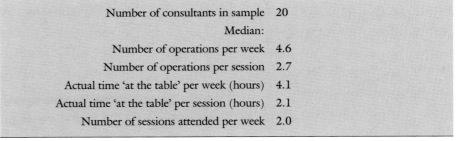

Number of consultants in sample	20
Median:	
Number of operations per week	4.6
Number of operations per session	2.7
Actual time 'at the table' per week (hours)	4.1
Actual time 'at the table' per session (hours)	2.1
Number of sessions attended per week	2.0

Note: Each bar represents one consultant. They are consistently ordered in each graph, based on case-mix-adjusted weekly output.

Source: Audit Commission.

Exhibit A4.5
Consultant surgeons' NHS operating theatre work

Urology

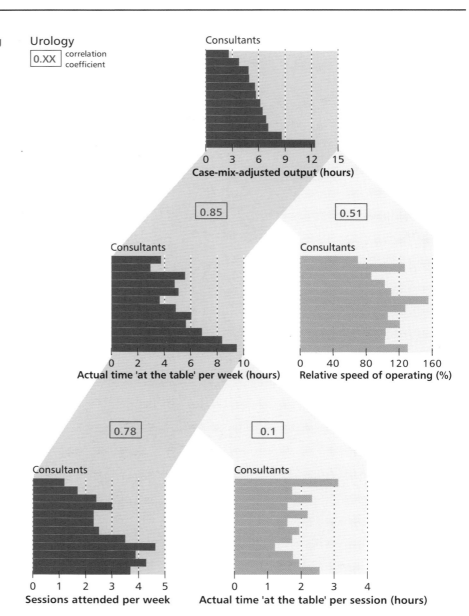

| | 0.XX | correlation coefficient |

Consultants

Case-mix-adjusted output (hours)

0.85   0.51

Consultants   Consultants

Actual time 'at the table' per week (hours)   Relative speed of operating (%)

0.78   0.1

Consultants   Consultants

Sessions attended per week   Actual time 'at the table' per session (hours)

Note: Each bar represents one consultant. They are consistently ordered in each graph, based on case-mix-adjusted weekly output.

Source: Audit Commission.

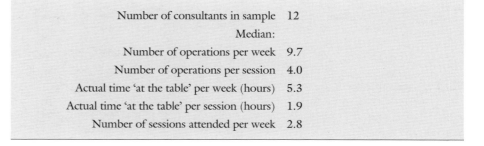

Number of consultants in sample	12
Median:	
Number of operations per week	9.7
Number of operations per session	4.0
Actual time 'at the table' per week (hours)	5.3
Actual time 'at the table' per session (hours)	1.9
Number of sessions attended per week	2.8

It can be argued that exclusion of the 'gap time' between each operation may bias the comparison of workload because actual time 'at the table' (used in the analysis) is likely to be proportionally greater for consultants who do fewer operations. In fact there is no evidence of this for any of the specialties included. On the contrary, in general surgery, for example, if anything, the evidence suggests that consultants who do more operations per session also tend to operate more hours at the operating table, but the relationship is not strong (Exhibit A4.6).

The data was also used to look at supervision of doctors in operating theatres during the day and at night. These results are presented in Exhibit 10, page 21, with additional data from pilot audit sites where available.

Exhibit A4.6
The relationship between operating hours (actual time 'at the table') and the number of operations

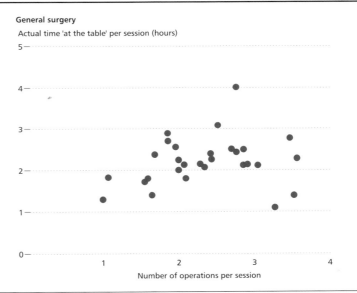

General surgery

Actual time 'at the table' per session (hours)

Number of operations per session

Sample size: 29 consultants.

Source: Audit Commission.

Appendix 5 – Comparison of NHS and Private Operating Theatre Work

NHS consultants are permitted to undertake private practice at any time as long as they *'devote substantially the whole of their professional time to the NHS'* (Ref. 23). This raises the issue of whether there is any relationship between the quantity of consultants' NHS work and the quantity of their private work. Is private work done at the expense of NHS work? In order to answer this question data on the type and amount of work carried out privately over the same period and involving the same full-time consultants (141 surgeons and 86 anaesthetists) as in the Audit Commission's sample of work in NHS operating theatres (Appendix 4) was obtained from a number of private sector insurers. This included private work at both NHS and private hospitals. The case-mix-adjusted weekly outputs of individual consultants in the NHS and private sector were calculated using the weights in table A4.1 (page 74) and were matched by an independent academic research group using anonymous identifying codes to ensure complete confidentiality of the individuals involved.

The distributions of NHS and private work amongst surgeons differ markedly within and between specialties (Exhibit A5.1). A simple scatter plot or correlation between all consultants would not therefore be valid. Instead, the number of consultants above and below the upper quartile of private work and above and below the lower quartile of NHS work were recorded in a two-way contingency table, separately for each of the five main surgical specialties in the sample and anaesthetics, and for the remaining smaller specialties combined. The numbers in these ranges were then summed to produce a table for all the

Exhibit A5.1
NHS and private operations

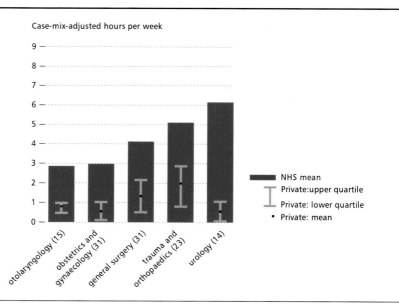

Case-mix-adjusted hours per week

Note: The number of consultants in each case is given in brackets after the specialty name.

Source: Audit Commission.

specialties combined. The expected number of doctors was also calculated for each cell in the table, assuming that private and NHS workloads were independent of one another.

For the majority of consultants no overall relationship is discernible. However, there is a statistically significant tendency for there to be more doctors in the 'high private/low NHS' categories than one would expect ($p < 0.01$, using chi-square, Exhibit A5.2).

Exhibit A5.2
Comparison of high private and low NHS workloads

Number of consultants doing:	less than the upper quartile of private work	more than the upper quartile of private work	Total
less than the lower quartile of NHS work	37 (44.41)	19 (11.59)	56
more than the lower quartile of NHS work	143 (135.59)	28 (35.41)	171
Total	180	47	227

Numbers are actual frequencies with expected frequencies (assuming NHS and private work are independent) in brackets.

Chi-square = 7.93 at 1 degree of freedom, $p < 0.01$

Source: Audit Commission.

Appendix 6 – Consultants' NHS Outpatient Work

The data on outpatient clinics was collected from the pilot audit sites. The data obtained included: number of consultations, grades of doctors attending and attendance times of consultants. The data was collected over a five- or six-week period during April to June 1994, avoiding public holidays.

The measure of output used for the analysis of consultants' work is the number of outpatients seen by each consultant per week. The data has not been adjusted for case complexity and so this measure will be affected by sub-specialty differences in average case complexity. In most specialties it is determined more by consultants' attendance rates than their speed of working (Exhibits A6.1 to A6.3).

Exhibit A6.1
Consultants' work in outpatient clinics

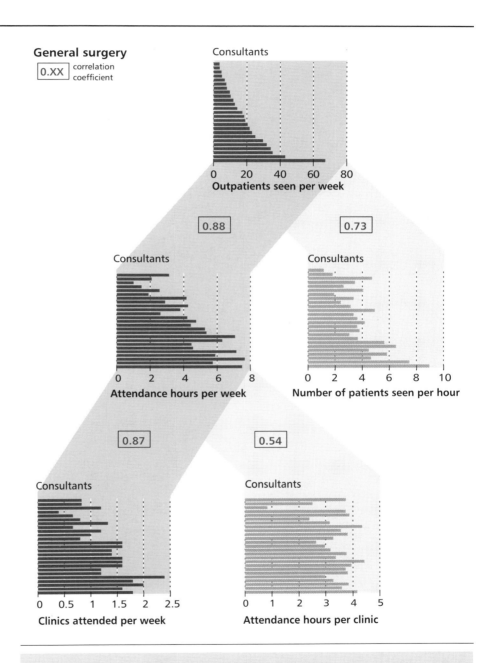

General surgery

| 0.XX | correlation coefficient |

Note: Each bar represents one consultant. They are consistently ordered in each graph, based on outpatients seen per week.

Source: Audit Commission.

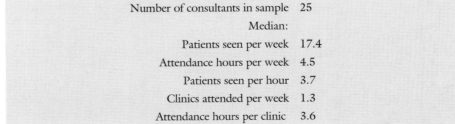

Number of consultants in sample	25
Median:	
Patients seen per week	17.4
Attendance hours per week	4.5
Patients seen per hour	3.7
Clinics attended per week	1.3
Attendance hours per clinic	3.6

Exhibit A6.2
Consultants' work in outpatient clinics

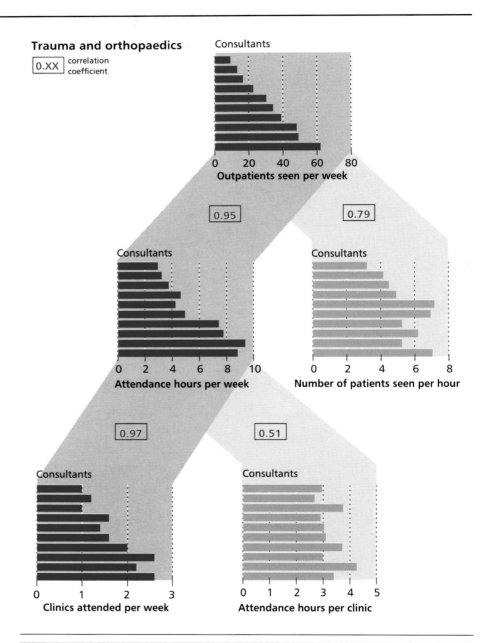

Trauma and orthopaedics

0.XX correlation coefficient

Consultants

Outpatients seen per week

0.95

0.79

Consultants — Attendance hours per week

Consultants — Number of patients seen per hour

0.97

0.51

Consultants — Clinics attended per week

Consultants — Attendance hours per clinic

Note: Each bar represents one consultant. They are consistently ordered in each graph, based on outpatients seen per week.

Source: Audit Commission.

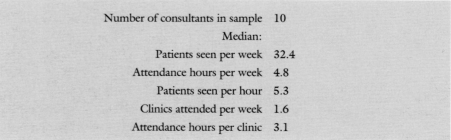

Number of consultants in sample	10
Median:	
Patients seen per week	32.4
Attendance hours per week	4.8
Patients seen per hour	5.3
Clinics attended per week	1.6
Attendance hours per clinic	3.1

Exhibit A6.3
Consultants' work in outpatient
clinics

General medicine

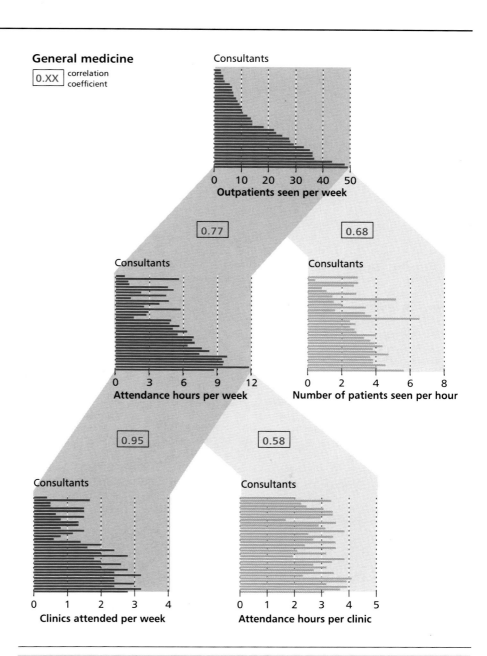

Note: Each bar represents one consultant.
They are consistently ordered in each graph,
based on out-patients seen per week.

Source: Audit Commission.

Number of consultants in sample	35
Median:	
Patients seen per week	13.4
Attendance hours per week	5.5
Patients seen per hour	3.4
Clinics attended per week	1.7
Attendance hours per clinic	3.2

References

1. Ian Morrison and Richard Smith (1994), The Future of Medicine, *British Medical Journal,* vol. 309, pp. 1099-1110.

2. Isobel Allen (1988), *Doctors and Their Careers,* Policy Studies Institute.

3. Rosemary Stevens (1966), *Medical Practice in Modern England: The Impact of Specialisation and State Medicine,* Yale University Press.

4. Dr. Brian Mawhinney MP (1993), *Medical Staffing Policies, Address to the Harveian Society, 8th December,* Department of Health EL(94)13.

5. UK Health Departments, Joint Consultants' Committee and Chairmen of Regional Health Authorities (1987), *Hospital Medical Staffing: Achieving a Balance – Plan for Action,* Department of Health

6. NHS Management Executive (1994), *The New Deal: Plan for Action,* Department of Health EL(94)17.

7. Robin Dowie (1989), *Patterns of Hospital Medical Staffing, Interim Report, Junior Doctors Hours.* British Postgraduate Medical Federation, HMSO.

8. Review Body on Doctors' and Dentists' Remuneration (1994), *Twenty-Third Report* cm 2460, HMSO.

9. Department of Health (1993), *Hospital Doctors: Training for the Future, The Report of the Working Group on Specialist Medical Training (the Calman Report),* Department of Health.

10. Sue Dowling and Sue Barrett (1991), *Doctors in the Making: The Experience of the Pre-Registration Year,* School for Advanced Urban Studies, University of Bristol.

11. Department of Health (1994), *Changing Childbirth, Part 1: Report of the Expert Maternity Group,* HMSO.

12. Theresa M. Marteau, Geralyn Wynne, W. Kaye, T. R. Evans (1990), Resuscitation: Experience Without Feedback Increases Confidence but not Skill, *British Medical Journal,* vol. 300, pp. 849-850.

13. Martin McKee and Nick Black (1993), Junior Doctors' Work at Night: What is Done and How Much is Appropriate?, *Journal of Public Health Medicine,* vol. 15, no 1, pp. 16-24.

14. E. A. Campling, H. B. Devlin, R. W. Hoile, J. N. Lunn (1993), *The Report of the National Enquiry into Perioperative Deaths 1991/1992,* Royal College of Surgeons of England.

15. Robin Dowie (1991), *Patterns of Hospital Medical Staffing, Specialty Reports for: Paediatrics, Obstetrics and Gynaecology, General Surgery, Trauma and Orthopaedic Surgery, Ophthalmology, Anaesthetics, General Medicine,* British Post Graduate Medical Federation, HMSO.

16. Isobel Allen (1994), *Doctors and their Careers: A New Generation,* Policy Studies Institute.

17. Standing Committee on Postgraduate Medical and Dental Education (SCOPME, 1994), *Meeting the Educational Needs of Staff Grade Doctors and Dentists,* SCOPME.

18. Susanne Holmes (1993), Is There a Future for Cardiac Surgeon Assistants in Britain, *New Deal News,* March, NHS Management Executive.

19. Yvonne Bell (editor) (1993), *The New Deal Tool Kit,* Oxford Regional Task Force, Oxford Regional Health Authority.

20. Martin McKee and Nick Black (1992), Does the Current Use of Junior Doctors in the United Kingdom Affect the Quality of Medical Care?, *Social Science and Medicine,* vol. 34, no 4, pp. 549-558.

21. Review Body on Doctors and Dentists Remuneration (1990), *Twentieth Report,* cm 937, HMSO.

22. Robin Dowie (1991), *Patterns of Hospital Medical Staffing: Overview,* British Postgraduate Medical Federation, HMSO.

23. Department of Health and Welsh Office (1994), *Hospital Medical and Dental Staff (England and Wales), Terms and Conditions of Service,* Department of Health.

24. Department of Health (1990), *Consultants' Contracts and Job Plans,* HC(90)16, Department of Health.

25. Royal College of Surgeons of England (1990), *Model Job Description for Consultant Posts in General Surgery: General Notes for Guidance.*

26. Monopolies and Mergers Commission (1993), *Private Medical Services,* HMSO.

27. Liam J. Donaldson (1994), Doctors with Problems in the NHS Workforce, *British Medical Journal,* vol. 308, pp. 1277-1282.

28. Herbert J. J. M. Berden, Frank F. Williams, Jo M. A. Hendrick, Nico H. J. Pijls, Johannes T. A. Knape (1993), How Frequently Should Basic Cardio Pulmonary Resuscitation Training be Repeated to Maintain Adequate Skills?, *British Medical Journal,* vol. 306, pp. 1576-1577.

29 NHS Management Executive (1993), *Flexible Training: Career Registrars,* HSG(93)52.

30. NHS Management Executive (1994), *Introduction of Compulsory Induction Courses and Changing the Starting Date for Hospital Medical and Dental Staff,* EL(94)1 and EL(94)44.

31. Royal College of Ophthalmologists (1993), *Record of Basic Specialist Training for Senior House Officers in Ophthalmology.*

32. NHS Management Executive (1993), *Report of the Joint Working Party on Flexible Training,* EL(93)49.

33. NHS Executive (1994), *Implementation of the Report of the Working Group on Specialist Medical Training – 'Hospital Doctors: Training for the Future,'* EL(94)71.

34. National Association of Health Authorities and Trusts (1994), *Approaches to Pay and Reward by NHS Trusts.*

35. Advisory Committee on Distinction Awards (1994), *First Annual Report,* Department of Health.

36. Department of Health (1994), *Report of the Working Party on the Review of the Consultants' Distinction Awards Scheme,* Department of Health.

37. British Association of Medical Managers, British Medical Association, The Institute of Health Services Management and the Royal College of Nursing (1993), *Managing Clinical Services: A Consensus Statement of Principles for Effective Clinical Management,* Institute of Health Services Management.

38. The Senate of the Royal Surgical Colleges of Great Britain and Ireland (1994), *Consultant Practice and Surgical Training in the United Kingdom.*

Index *References are to paragraph numbers*

Achieving a Balance 20-1, 84

Apprenticeship model of training 24, 25

Calman Report 24, 84, 92

Cardio-pulmonary resuscitation (CPR) 32, 86

Career advice 37, 56, 57

Career progression 11, 32, 55

Certificate of Completion of Specialist Training (CCST) 24

Changes in health care 2-5, 7, 15-17

Clinical directors 80, 104-106

Clinical nurse specialists 28

Clinical skills, assessment 85-86

Continuing medical education 96

Consultants

    annual review 80

    commitments 64-68, 76, 77

    contracts 64, 65

    distinction awards 103

    emergency patients 48, 50

    'firms' 25, 26

    job plans 64-67, 74-80

    junior doctors' access to 46

    monitoring 78-9

    non-clinical duties 63, 66

    patient allocation between 48

    planned growth in numbers of 21

    professional development 95

    role in service and training 61

    support staff 20

    surgery analysis 69

    surveys of activity 66-73

    team working between 48

    'ten per cent-of-income' rule 79

    work loads 33, 53, 68-73, 81

    work in operating theatres 69

    work in out-patient clinics 70

    work patterns 62

    see also Private practice; Referral system

Continuing professional development 89, 95-96

Day cases 15

Disease management 17

Disease patterns 16

Distinction awards 103

Doctors' mess 39

ECG technicians 28

Educational supervisor 85

Emergencies

    distribution between consultants 48

    junior doctors in 30

    timing of surgery 34

Emergency cover 25, 36, 37, 50, 51

    accommodation needs 39

    duties required during 35

    number of tiers in rotas 36, 53

    specialties 54

Emergency referrals 35, 50

Emergency work load 13, 48

Employment opportunities and support 55-58

Family commitments 37, 38, 55

'Firms' 25, 26

Handover arrangements 52

Health care, changing demand 2-5, 7, 15-17

Hospital doctors

    allocation of tasks and supervision 44-47

    availability for patient care 17

    changes in grade structure 21

    changing supply of 18

    definition of roles in relation to other professions 41-43

    deployment according to demand 50-54

    distribution by specialty 12

    grades and their roles 25

    involvement in management 104

    job descriptions 28, 44-47

    lack of support 37-40

    responsibilities 4, 5

    role of 1

    statistics 10

    work organisation 98

Hospital nurses, changing role of 28

Hospital patients, length of stay 17

Hospital trusts 3

    primary role 27

Hours of work of junior doctors 22-3, 25, 28, 36, 41, 47

House officers 47

Incentives 101-103

Induction training 85

In-patients 15

Job descriptions 28, 44-47

Job satisfaction 58

Job sharing 57

Junior doctors

    access to consultant 46

    assessment of skills 32

    changing role of 28

    hours of work 22-3, 25, 28, 36, 41, 47

in emergencies   30

inappropriate tasks undertaken by   28

information leaflet   91

insufficient supervision   29-32

model contents of handbook   90

Management process   104-107

Management structure   104

Managers

relationship with doctors   107

role of   6

Medical intervention   17

Medical staffing

government initiatives   18

levels of   35

local structure   25-26

national controls   100

national policy   19

new professional roles   41-43

number of tiers in rotas   36

recommendations on skill mix and deployment   59-60

workload   35

Medical technology   2, 17

Midwives   28

National Confidential Enquiry into Peri-operative Deaths   34

New Deal   22-3, 39, 50, 58, 84

New technology   2, 17

Nurse practitioners   28

On-call emergency cover. *See* Emergency cover

Operating theatres   34

supervision of juniors in   30

time-tables   49

use by consultants   69

Outmoded practices   7

Out-of-hours cover. *See* Emergency cover

Out-patient clinics   34

supervision of juniors in   30-31

time-tables   49

use by consultants   70

Part-time career posts   37

Part-time training   87, 94

Part-time work   57

Patient focused care   42

Phlebotomists   28

Population statistics   16

Postgraduate training   24, 82, 85-86

management   90-91

purchaser/provider split   90

strategy implementation   90

structures   87

Private practice   62, 71-73

Professional development   89

Referral system   33, 48, 71

Rota systems   36, 51, 52

Senior house officers (SHOs), insufficient supervision   30

Shift and partial-shift systems   50-52

Specialist

definition   24

re-certification   96

Specialties

emergency cover   54

joint working   54

Specialty groupings   12-13, 17

Study leave   89, 95

Surgeons' assistants   28

Training   10, 11, 18, 27, 82

apprenticeship model   24, 25

assessment and appraisal   85-86

changes in conduct of   84

curricula   24

flexibility needs   38, 88, 92

major changes in direction   24

new combinations of knowledge and skills   43

organisation   83

part-time   87, 94

programmes   85, 92

quality and quantity   51

standards and policies   84

structured approach   87, 92

uncoordinated   93

Women doctors   37, 38, 56

Women in Surgical Training (WIST)   56

Working practices   5, 25, 26